Renal Diet Cookbook

The Complete Guide To Avoid Dialysis, Low Sodium, Low Potassium, Low Phosphorous

Susan Moore

**© Copyright 2019 by Susan Moore
All rights reserved.**

This document is geared towards providing exact and reliable information with regards to the topic and issue covered. The publication is sold with the idea that the publisher is not required to render accounting, officially permitted, or otherwise, qualified services. If advice is necessary, legal or professional, a practiced individual in the profession should be ordered.

- From a Declaration of Principles which was accepted and approved equally by a Committee of the American Bar Association and a Committee of Publishers and Associations.

In no way is it legal to reproduce, duplicate, or transmit any part of this document in either electronic means or in printed format. Recording of this publication is strictly prohibited and any storage of this document is not allowed unless with written permission from the publisher. All rights reserved.

The information provided herein is stated to be truthful and consistent, in that any liability, in terms of inattention or otherwise, by any usage or abuse of any policies, processes, or directions contained within is the solitary and utter responsibility of the recipient reader. Under no circumstances will any legal responsibility or blame be held against the publisher for any reparation, damages, or monetary loss due to the information herein, either directly or indirectly.

Respective authors own all copyrights not held by the publisher.

The information herein is offered for informational purposes solely, and is universal as so. The presentation of the information is without contract or any type of guarantee assurance.

The trademarks that are used are without any consent, and the publication of the trademark is without permission or backing by the trademark owner. All trademarks and brands within this book are for clarifying purposes only and are the owned by the owners themselves, not affiliated with this document

Contents

Introduction 1

Part 1 – Introduction to Kidney Disease . 3

What is Chronic Kidney Disease? 3

What are the causes of chronic kidney disease? 5

What are the symptoms of kidney disease? 8

What are the stages of kidney failure? 9

What are the treatments for kidney failure? 12

Part 2 – Living Healthy with Renal Diet 16

What is the renal diet? 16

Micronutrients for renal diet 17

What to eat and avoid on a renal diet? 23

Part 3 – Stocking for Pantry 32

Kidney-Friendly Kitchen Staples 32

BBQ Rub for Chicken 32

Cajun Seasoning 33

Chinese Five-Spice Blend 34

Taco Seasoning 35

Mexican Blend 36

Mixed Herb Blend 37

Poultry Seasoning 38

Fajita Flavor Marinade 39

Garlic-Herb Seasoning 40

Honey Mustard 41

Soy Sauce.. 42

Barbecue Sauce 43

Teriyaki Sauce.. 44

Pizza Sauce 45

Alfredo Sauce 46

Tomato Salsa 48

Basil Oil... 49

Ranch Dressing 50

Turkey Broth.. 52

Pickles... 53

Part 5 – Meal Planning For Renal Diet . 55

30-Day Meal Plan 55

Week 1 55

Day 1.. 55

Day 2.. 55

Day 3.. 56

Day 4.. 56

Day 5.. 56

Day 6.. 57

Day 7 57
Week 2 57
Day 8 57
Day 9 58
Day 10 58
Day 11 58
Day 12 59
Day 13 59
Day 14 59

Week 3 60
Day 15 60
Day 16 60
Day 17 60
Day 18 61
Day 19 61
Day 20 61
Day 21 62

Week 4 62
Day 22 62
Day 23 62
Day 24 63
Day 25 63

- Day 26 63
- Day 27 64
- Day 28 64

Week 5 64

- Day 29 64
- Day 30 65
- Week 1 Shopping List 66
- Week 2 Shopping List 71
- Week 3 Shopping List 77
- Week 4 Shopping List 83

Part 6 – Recipes 88

- Breakfast 88
- Lemon Apple Honey Smoothie 88
- Banana Oat Shake 89
- Banana and Apple Smoothie 90
- "Berrylicious" Smoothie 91
- Fruit Lassi 92
- Gingersnap Cookies 93
- Omelet 94
- Southern-style Cornbread 95
- Breakfast Burrito 97
- Vegetables Omelet 98

Fruity Dump Cake 100
Short Bread Cookies 101
Bagel with Egg and Salmon 102
Berry Smoothie Bowl 103
Apple and Onion Omelet 104
Asparagus and Cauliflower Tortilla 106
Clam Omelet 108
Cheese Pancakes with Strawberries 109
Cottage Cheese and Sour Cream Pancakes 110
Egg and Sausage Breakfast Sandwich 111
Stuffed French Toast 112
Corn Cakes with Cheese 114
Potato Gratin 115
Old Fashion Waffles 116
Spaghetti-Basil Frittata 118
Strawberry and Cream Cheese French Toast Casserole 119
Wheat and Berry Breakfast Bowl 121
Cranberry and Roasted Garlic Risotto 123
Zucchini Frittata 124
Zucchini Pancakes 126
Lunch 128
Deviled Green Beans 128

Cranberry Cabbage	129
Buffalo Chicken Dip	130
Tortilla Pizza	131
Vegetarian Pizza	133
Chiles Rellenos	134
Pasta Primavera	136
Tempeh Pita Sandwiches	137
Triple Berry Salad	138
Veggie Strata	139
Buffalo Wings	142
Mashed Cauliflower Potatoes	143
Potato Salad	144
Flavorful Grilled Salmon	146
Salmon and Summer Squash	147
Autumn Wild Rice	149
Gratin Pasta with Chicken and Watercress	151
Cranberry Rice Pilaf	152
Lemon Rice with Vegetables	153
Singapore Rice Noodles	155
Shrimp Fried Rice	157
Grilled Salmon Sandwiches	158
Shrimp and Broccoli Fettuccine	160
Fish Fry with Seasoned Rice	162

Korean-Style Fried Fish	163
Pumpkin Chili	165
Chicken Noodle Soup	166
Crab Cakes	167
Eggplant Seafood Casserole	169
Seafood Corn Chowder	171
Dinner	173
Chicken Chili	173
Chicken Wild Rice Soup	174
Cauliflower Manchurian	176
Ratatouille	177
Roasted Brussels Sprouts, Carrots and Apples	179
Chicken Lettuce Wraps	180
Chicken Parmesan Meatballs	182
Mexican Chicken Pizza	183
Pita Pizza	185
Tofu Stir Fry	187
Mediterranean Pizza	189
Penne Pasta with Asparagus	190
Vegetarian Egg Fried Rice	191
Vegetable Casserole Delight	193
Macaroni and Cheese	194
Salmon Burgers with Coleslaw	195

Honey Mustard Grilled Chicken 197

Broiled Haddock with Cucumber Salsa 198

Citrus Salmon 200

Honey Spice-Rubbed Salmon 201

Salmon Soup.. 203

Salmon Steaks with Herb Dressing............................ 204

Tuna Noodle Casserole.. 206

Glazed Cornish Game Hen.. 207

Cauliflower and Broccoli Mac-n-Cheese 209

Creamy Orzo and Vegetables 211

Feta Pasta with Chicken and Asparagus.................... 213

Creamy Shells with Peas and Bacon.......................... 215

Hawaiian Rice 217

Italian Style Vegetables and Pasta with Chicken....... 218

Dessert 220

Berry Galette 220

Berries Napoleon... 221

Banana Dessert 222

Crepes with Frozen Berries 224

Carrot Cake.. 225

Stuffed Strawberries 227

Sugarless Heart Cookies 228

Low Phosphorus Fudge 229

- Cherry Coffee Cake 231
- Cranberry and Apple Salad 232
- Creamy Grape Salad 233
- Orange Pineapple Ambrosia Salad 234
- Caramel Custard 235
- Pear Crisp... 237
- Dessert Pizza.. 238
- Something Extra – Snacks and Juices 240
- Rhubarb Tea 240
- Lemonade.. 241
- Ginger and Cranberry Punch 242
- Raspberry Punch.. 243
- Watermelon Summer Cooler 244
- Spiced Almonds and Cashews 245
- Sweet Potato Fries... 246
- Eggplant French Fries 247
- Zucchini French Fries... 248
- Thyme Corn on the Cob... 250

Conclusion 252

Introduction

Are you someone who is overwhelmed with the changes in lifestyle due to kidney disease? Your problem is solved with the amazing renal diet. But following a renal diet on your own can become another challenging aspect of your life. Not only you have to determine what foods are good or bad for you, you then have to come up with meals that are easy-to-prepare, satisfying to eat, and nutritious as well. This all requires in-depth knowledge about your body, its response during kidney diseases, and most importantly, guidelines for renal diet meal planning. We have compiled all this information for you in this cookbook.

You will find details of chronic kidney diseases, its causes and possible treatment, and how effectively you can live a healthy life with renal diet, without any stress. Moreover, we have also collected some essential kidney-friendly kitchen staples and tasty recipes that cover your next 30 days of meal planning. At the bottom of each recipe, you will find nutritional information to help you know the food and modifying the meals according to your personal needs. If you are not sure about the recipes, feel free to check it with your doctor or dietician.

Read on to know more.

Part 1 – Introduction to Kidney Disease

What is Chronic Kidney Disease?

The kidney plays a vital role in our body. Each kidney is of the size of a fist and located at the lowest level of the ribcage and either side of the spine. Kidneys contain a network of million functioning units called *nephrons*, which are consistent of tiny blood vessels called *glomeruli*. These blood vessels attached to a tubule and act as a filtering unit and thus, filtered the blood passing through them. The remaining fluid is passed along the tubule where water and chemicals are either removed or added as per body needs and product the urine, which our body excretes.

In other words, our kidneys are like powerful chemical factories that do 24-hours jobs of filtering and returning to the bloodstream. The major function of the kidneys is to remove excess fluid, waste products, and drugs from the body through the urine. This excretion process is necessary to maintain a stable balance of the body fluid and minerals and salts like calcium, sodium, potassium, and phosphorus. Without this balance of minerals and fluid in the body, the muscles, tissues, and nerves may not work correctly. The kidney also produces an active form of vitamin D that promotes healthy and strong bones. Moreover, the kidney also makes hormones that help in controlling metabolism, production of red blood cells, and regulating blood pressure.

When the kidneys are damaged and are unable to filter excess fluid and water products from the blood the way they should, this condition is called *Chronic Kidney Disease* (CKD). The kidney disease is called "chronic" because the loss of function and damage to the kidneys happens over a long period. This ultimately results in the accumulation of waste at dangerous levels. Along with this, CKD also causes other health conditions such as high blood pressure, diabetes, and heart disease.

What are the causes of chronic kidney disease?

Chronic kidney disease (CKD) occurs when a specific health condition or disease impairs the function of the kidney, which causes kidney damage to worsen for three months or longer. There are many causes of CKD. These include:

1- Diabetes – Diabetes occurs when the body cannot use insulin properly or fails to make enough insulin. High or low blood sugar levels due to diabetes can damage the blood vessels of the kidneys.
2- High blood pressure – Also known as hypertension, can also damage the blood vessels in kidneys. When hypertension is controlled, the risk of developing CKD and other health conditions like heart attack and stroke is decreased.
3- Heart disease – Individuals with heart diseases have a higher risk of developing CKD and vice versa. The longer you have heart disease, the more likely you are to suffer from chronic kidney disease.
4- Glomerulonephritis – This disease is caused by the inflammation of glomeruli. Although Glomerulonephritis may happen

all of a sudden and the patient may get well soon; but due to it, kidney disease may develop slowly, and after several years, it may cause loss of kidney function.

5- Polycystic kidney disease – It is the most common inherited kidney disease and is characterized by the enlargement of kidney cysts that happen over time. It causes severe kidney damage and at times, leads to failure of kidneys.

6- Family history of kidney failure – CKD runs in families; so, if your blood relation like parents or siblings has a history of kidney failure, you are at risk for chronic kidney disease.

7- Kidney stones – They are a very common cause of kidney disease. The leading causes of kidney stones can be an inherited disorder, urinary tract infections, or too much calcium in the food. Most of the time, proper diet and medication prevent recurrent stone formation, but when the stones are too large, they are either removed surgically or break down into small pieces so that they can pass out of the body. Its symptoms are severe pain in your back and sometimes in the side.

8- Urinary tract infections – Like any other infection, it occurs when germs enter the urinary tract. The symptoms include frequent urination, burning, or, pain during urination. The urinary tract infections affect the bladder, but they often spread to the kidneys and cause pain in the back and fever.
9- Congenital diseases –These diseases occu in the urinary tract during pregnancy. Due to congenital diseases, the valve-like mechanism between urine tube (ureter) and the bladder don't work correctly, which leads to back up of urine to the kidneys. And, this causes kidney infections and possible damage.
10- Drugs and toxins – If you frequently use over-the-counter pain killers, they may be harmful to the kidneys. Drugs like heroin, pesticides, toxins, and taking other medications over a long time also cause severe damage to the kidney.

Overall, you are at high risk for chronic kidney disease if you:

- Have diabetes
- Have heart disease
- Have high blood pressure

- Are elderly
- Have a family history of CKD
- Are a Pacific Islander, Asian, American Indian, African American, or Hispanic American

What are the symptoms of kidney disease?

As said before, CKD develops over time, so you may never know you have developed kidney disease because you feel fine. So, you can have kidney damage without any symptoms because your kidney will keep doing enough work to make you feel well. Therefore, you can't detect CKD at the early stage, except through urine tests or blood tests for kidneys. However, as the kidney disease grows worse, the patient may have swelling called edema. The swelling occurs in ankles, legs, and feet, sometimes on the face and in the hands. It happens when kidneys get failed to get rid of salt and extra fluid.

Some more symptoms are:

- weight loss
- loss of appetite
- nausea

- vomiting
- headaches
- muscle cramps
- feeling tired
- sleep problems
- shortness of breath
- dry skin
- itching or numbness
- chest pain
- trouble concentrating
- increased or decreased urination

Many people are afraid to get themselves tested for CKD because they don't want to learn that they have kidney disease and thus, keep delaying in consulting the doctor. However, the sooner you know you have CKD, the sooner you can make healthy changes in your lifestyle to protect your kidneys.

What are the stages of kidney failure?

The kidney failure is classified into five stages, and as the stages progress, the complications increase as well.

Stage 1:

Some damage is present in this stage, but the patient may not experience any symptoms, and neither are there any visible complications. Therefore, this is a mild stage, and there could be a possibility for the patient to manage kidney disease and make progress towards the sustained health of kidneys. This will include eating a healthy balanced diet, regular workout, maintaining a healthy weight, and not using tobacco products.

Stage 2:

The physical damage to the kidneys may become more obvious in this stage, and the disease could be detected through urine and blood test. A healthy lifestyle approach that helped in stage 1 of CKD should be used in stage 2 as well for treatment. Along with it, discuss this situation with a doctor and talk about other factors that could speed up kidney failures such as inflammation, blood pressure, and heart disease.

Stage 3:

This is a moderate stage of kidney disease. The kidneys aren't working as they should be and the symptoms become more apparent, such as; swelling, back pain, frequent urination, etc.

Usually, a blood test is performed to measure out the level of waste in the body. A healthy lifestyle approach helps, but medications also become essential to treat the conditions that may contribute to kidney failure.

Stage 4:

The kidneys aren't working well in this stage, but there isn't a danger of kidney failure yet. The patient feels symptoms, including high blood pressure, anemia, bone disease, etc. Maintaining a healthy lifestyle becomes vital, and the doctors will design a proper treatment plan to slow the damage.

Stage 5:

Stage 5 or advanced stage of kidney disease leads to complete failure. When this happens, the patient will need a kidney transplant or dialysis to maintain the health. The symptoms of impaired kidney function will become evident, including itchy skin, nausea, vomiting, trouble breathing, and more.

What are the treatments for kidney failure?

The treatment for kidney failure depends on its type.

1- Dialysis
   When kidneys fail to do their job of removing excess fluids and toxins from the blood, dialysis then replaces kidneys to perform this function. It is done by a machine that filters and purifies the blood and maintains the balance of fluid and electrolytes. It doesn't cure kidney failure, but it surely extends your life if you have it regularly.

   There are three types of dialysis:

   Hemodialysis – It involves the use of an artificial kidney to remove extra water and waste from the blood. The blood from the body is transferred to an artificial kidney where it is filtered through, and then purified blood is returned to the body. This dialysis treatment takes three to five hours and usually performed three times a week. The time of treatment depends on the amount of waste in the blood, size of body, and state of health.

Peritoneal dialysis – This treatment involves the surgical implantation of a catheter into the abdomen. The catheter contains a special fluid called dialysate, which absorbs waste from the blood and then drains it from the abdomen. The process of this treatment lasts a few hours and needs to be done three to six times a day.

Hemofiltration – this treatment is focused on patients with acute kidney failure, primarily in intensive care. A dialysis machine passes the blood and filter water and waste products through the tubing, and then the blood is returned into the body. This procedure is performed one to twenty-four times in a day, and generally every day.

2- Kidney transplant
Another option for the treatment of kidney failure is a kidney transplant. If your body qualifies for a kidney transplant, then there is no need to be dependent on

dialysis treatment. Surgery is performed on the patient, which results in the replacement of one or both failed kidneys with the donor's kidneys, either from a deceased or live person. A donor can be a healthy person from your family or someone who has a similar blood group. If there is no in a family member whose kidney matches with you, a deceased donor can be your potential option. A deceased donor can be anyone who has died in an accident rather than a disease, and their family has given consent to donate his/her organ. If your tissues matched with the deceased donor's and passed the anti-body test, you can use the new kidney in place of your failed ones. After the surgery, you will live an active life, but you will have to take immune-suppressing drugs to keep your immune system away from attacking your new kidney.

3- Kidney friendly diet

   As mentioned before, maintaining a healthy lifestyle routine is vital to treat kidney disease and kidney failure. But what you should eat depends on the stage of your kidney disease and your current health. Overall, your diet should have fewer minerals, such as sodium, potassium, and phosphorus. You need to aim to eat less than 2000 mg sodium and potassium in a day. Stay below 1000 mg per day when you are eating phosphorus. Moreover, you will also have to cut back protein in your early or moderate stage of CKD. However, your doctor may recommend you eat more protein in the end stage of kidney disease or kidney failure.

Read more about a kidney-friendly diet in the next section.

Part 2 – Living Healthy with Renal Diet

What is the renal diet?

People with compromised kidneys or kidney failure are recommended to adhere to a kidney-friendly or renal diet. The renal diet emphasizes removing waste from the blood by reducing the consumption of protein, fluid, sodium, potassium, and phosphorus. This diet also focuses on promoting the eating of high-quality protein. The rationale behind these limitations is to prevent the building of macronutrients and minerals in the blood and reduce the complications of kidney diseases like fluid overload, blood pressure, bone disorder, arrhythmias, and vascular calcifications.

By following a renal diet, you can help in promoting the health of your kidneys and their function and slow the progress of kidney failure through food. The renal diet restricts some food groups in the diet such as vegetables, fruits, grains, nuts, legumes, and red meats that are high in salt and sugar.

Some people may limit sodium only, and some may restrict potassium as well. Every person is different; therefore, a patient with kidney disease has to work together with his dietician to tailor the renal diet that works well for him and cater to his needs.

Micronutrients for renal diet

The following are some substances that are essential to monitoring during the renal diet.

Sodium

Sodium is naturally found in every food. Most people take sodium and salt as interchangeable; however, salt is a compound of sodium and chloride.

Sodium helps in

- Regulating blood volume and pressure
- Regulating muscle contraction
- Regulating nerve function
- Balance acid in the blood
- Balance the fluid level in the body

Foods may also contain sodium in other forms; for example, foods that are processed have a higher level of sodium due to additional salt in them. Too much salt is harmful to people with kidney disease because, in this condition, the kidney couldn't properly eliminate excess sodium from the body. So, the level of sodium builds up and causes:

- Increased thirst
- Swelling in legs, feet, face, and hands
- High blood pressure
- Heart failure
- Shortness of breath

You can reduce sodium intake by:

- Limiting sodium intake to 140 mg per serving or 400 mg per meal
- Reading sodium content in the food or ingredients labels
- Paying close attention to sodium amount per serving size
- Consuming fresh meat, rather than packed ones
- Choosing fresh vegetables and fruits
- Selecting no-salt-added or low-sodium canned and frozen food items
- Avoiding processed foods

- Avoiding salt substitutes
- Cooking more at home, season food with own spices and herbs, and do not add salt
- Avoid medicines which contain sodium

Potassium

Potassium is naturally found in the body, and in many foods we eat. It keeps our muscles working correctly, and the heart beating regularly. It is also vital for maintaining electrolyte balance and fluid levels in the blood. The kidney plays a crucial role in keeping the potassium level in our body at the right level and excrete its excess amount into the urine.

When a kidney fails to function normally, it cannot remove extra potassium, and its level builds up in the blood and leads to a condition called hyperkalemia. Its signs are:

- Slow pulse
- Abnormal heartbeat
- Heart attack
- Weaken muscles
- Death

The following are some tips for the kidney disease patient for monitoring the amount of potassium in the body

- Read potassium content on the labels of packaged foods
- Restrict foods that are high in potassium
- Limit dairy products and milk to 8-ounce per day
- Consume fresh vegetables and fruits
- Avoid potassium chloride
- Keep a food journal

Phosphorus

Phosphorous is a critical micronutrient for maintaining bone development and health. It also assists in muscle movement, growth of organs, and connective tissue. When food is digested in the small intestine, it absorbs the phosphorus so that it can then be stored in the bones.

When your kidney can no longer work normally, it cannot remove extra phosphorus from the blood. The high level of phosphorus in the blood results in pulling calcium from the bones and hence, makes them weak. This could lead to a reduction of calcium to a dangerous level or the deposit of calcium in the eyes, lungs, heart, and blood vessels.

Here are the following tips that can help you managing phosphorus level in the body:

- Limit the foods that are high in protein (fresh meat contains 7 gm of protein and 65 mg of phosphorus per ounce)
- Eat high quality and low-fat protein
- Look for the prefix "PHOS" on the nutrition label of foods
- Avoid packaged and processed foods that contain added phosphorus
- Know what foods are low in phosphorus
- Eat fresh vegetables and fruits
- Take prescription of using phosphate binders during meal

Protein

When protein is digested, it is converted into amino acid and other proteins byproducts. It is essential for the maintenance of tissues and performing other body functions. Normally, nephrons in the kidney filtered out excess protein products, and with the addition of renal protein, all the waste products are turned into urine. In contrast, failed kidneys are unable to remove excess protein waste, and it builds up in the blood.

It is tricky to find out the proper consumption of protein for a kidney disease patient as the amount of protein differs from the stage of the disease.

Therefore, it is essential to follow your renal dietician or doctor guidelines for eating protein for the specific stage of the disease.

Fluids

Controlling fluid levels in the body is critical for the patients' kidney disease at a moderate or advanced stage because the high level of fluid in the body could become dangerous. People who are treated with dialysis have decreased urination, so taking more fluid could add additional pressure on the heart and lungs of that person.

The estimation of fluid intake depends on the individual, dialysis type, and urine output. Therefore, it is vital to follow your doctor's guideline for fluid intake. To help more with controlling fluid intake, you should:

- Avoid spicy foods
- Avoid soy sauce and other condiments
- Stay cool
- Not drink what your dietician or doctor have recommended
- Drink cold beverages
- Use small cups for sipping beverages
- Take medications with small sips of water

- Fluids also include those foods that melt at room temperature
- Take care about the amount of liquid used in cooking
- Maintain a food journal with daily fluid updates and also, add your weight

What to eat and avoid on a renal diet?

High sodium foods that people with CKD should avoid	Low-sodium foods to choose for people with CKD
Meat, sausage, poultry, ham, bacon, cold cuts that are salted, canned, smoked, breaded or cured	Cuts of poultry, lamb, beef, pork, fish and shrimps that are fresh or frozen
Fish, sardines, and anchovies that are salted, canned	Fish or poultry that is water or oil-packed and drained Low-sodium canned fish
Frozen dinners, such as pizza	
Canned food items like ravioli, chili, etc.	Eggs Egg substitutes
Salted nuts	Dry peas

Canned beans with additional-salt	Beans (not canned)
Buttermilk	Low-sodium peanut butter Almond milk, rice milk, coconut milk Soy-based yogurt or plant-based yogurt
Processed cheese, cheese spreads	Low-sodium cream cheese
Processed cottage cheese	Low-sodium cheeses, like parmesan cheese, ricotta cheese, mozzarella
Bread and quick breads with additional salt	Ready-to-eat cereals
Rolls with salted tops	Rolls, bagels, and breads without salted tops
Processed mixes of biscuit, pancake, and waffle with self-rising flour	Almond flour, coconut flour, whole-wheat flour, low-sodium plain, and all-purpose white flour Low-sodium corn Low-sodium flour tortillas
Salted crackers and croutons	Low sodium breadsticks Low-sodium crackers

	Unsalted popcorn and pretzels
Unsalted chips
Processed and prepackaged mixes for potatoes, rice, and pasta	All rice and pasta cooked without salt
Low-sodium noodles and pasta
Canned vegetables	Fresh and frozen vegetables, low-sodium canned vegetables, without sauces
Canned vegetable juices	Low-sodium vegetable juices
V-8 juice
Low-salt tomato juice
Regular salted pickles	Low-sodium pickles
Pickled olives, and other pickled vegetables	
Vegetables made with salted bacon, pork, ham	Fresh potatoes, frozen French fries without salt and seasoning, and instant mashed potatoes
Packaged and processed mixes, such as frozen hash browns, and scalloped potatoes	Fresh, frozen and canned fruit
Ready to eat pasta dinner	Dried fruits
Processed tomato sauces	

Processed salsa	Low-sodium salsa
Regular, dehydrated or canned soup, and bouillon	Low-sodium canned and dehydrated soups, and bouillon Soups cooked in the home with fresh ingredients and without added salt
Regular and processed broth	Homemade broth without salt
Packed cup of noodles	Home-cooked pasta without salt
Processed and seasoned ramen mixes	
Soy sauce	Low-sodium soy sauce and vinegar
Seasoning salt	Low-sodium seasoning and rubs
Salted marinades	Low-sodium marinades
Processed and regular bottled salad dressings	Low sodium salad dressings
Salad dressing with bacon bits	Low-sodium mayonnaise
Salted butter or margarine	Unsalted butter or margarine Vegetable oils
Instant pudding	All desserts made without salt
Ready to eat cake	

Processed tomato ketchup	Low-sodium and homemade tomato ketchup
Processed mustard with additional salt	Mustard without salt

High-potassium foods that people with CKD should avoid	**Low-potassium foods to choose for people with CKD**
Cooked spinach, tomato, artichokes, okra, cooked broccoli, beets, fried onions, sweet and white potato	Asparagus, kale, cabbage, broccoli, carrot, cucumber, zucchini, yellow squash, garlic, bell peppers, eggplant, lettuce
Bananas, avocado, honeydew, cantaloupe, Mango, orange, pomegranate, prune, pumpkins, coconut	Apple, grape, pineapple, watermelon and all berries, watermelon, peaches, plums
Buttermilk, milkshakes	Rice milk
Beans like baked and refried beans, and legumes such as lentils	Green beans, wax beans, snow peas
Whole grains and bran	White rice, bread (not whole-grain)
Nuts like walnuts and raisins	Dried cranberries

Granola	Unsalted popcorns and pretzels
Salty foods and fast foods like French fries	Hash browns and mashed potatoes made with leached potatoes
Processed meats like hot dogs	
Vegetable juices	Unsalted tomato juice, V8-juice
Salted sauces like tomato sauce and tomato paste	Apple sauce and unsalted sauces
Fruit juice like orange juice, pomegranate, prune juice	Apple juice, grape juice, pineapple juice, fruit cocktail
Creamed soup	Noodles and pasta without salt
Yogurt, frozen yogurt	Non-dairy creamer,
Ice cream	Sherbet
Chocolate desserts	Lemon or vanilla flavored desserts

Low-phosphorous foods to choose for people with CKD	
Vegetables	Baby carrots, celery, radish

Fruits	Apple, blueberries, strawberries, cherries, peach, pineapple,
Meat	Pot roast beef, sirloin steak
Poultry	Skinless chicken breast and chicken thighs, skinless turkey breast and thigh
Pork	Porkchop, hamburger patty (90% lean), pork roast
Game	Veal chop
Seafood	Wild-caught salmon, mahi-mahi, fresh and canned tuna (oil or water-packed), shrimp, oyster, snow crab, king crab, lobster
Bread	Plain bread without salted top, cinnamon bread, blueberry bread, sourdough bread, white bread, flatbread, Italian bread, light wheat bread, pita bread
Tortilla	Flour tortilla, corn tortilla
Muffin	English muffin

Pasta	Macaroni, egg noodle, rice noodles, spaghetti
Rice	Couscous, long-grain white rice,
Cheese	Cottage cheese, blue cheese, feta cheese, parmesan cheese, cream cheese
Milk	Almond milk, soya milk, rice milk,
Yogurt	Non-dairy creamer and whipped topping
Ice cream	Sorbet
Eggs	Pasteurized egg whites
Snack	Low-sodium crackers, unsalted popcorn, and pretzels

Kidney-Friendly Protein Foods
Burgers made with lean beef and turkey
Meat substitutes such as tofu, veggie sausage, and veggie burger
Skinless chicken breast and thighs
Salmon, trout, mackerel, shrimps
Pork chops
Cottage cheese
Pasteurized eggs
Greek yogurt

Milkshakes made with low-sodium milk such rice milk and almond milk

Kidney-friendly fluids
Fruits such as berries, apples, cherries, grapes, peaches, pears, zucchini
Vegetables such as broccoli, cabbage, cauliflower, carrot, celery, cucumber, eggplant, lettuce, bell peppers, pineapple, plums, tangerines
Tea
Coffee
Gelatin
Ice cubes
Popsicles
Fruit juice
Milk and milk substitute
Sherbet
Low-sodium soups

Part 3 – Stocking for Pantry

Kidney-Friendly Kitchen Staples

BBQ Rub for Chicken

|Preparation Time: 5 minutes|

|Cooking Time: 0 minutes|

|Total Time: 5 minutes|

|Serve – 3 tablespoons, 0.75 tablespoons per serving|

|Ingredients|

- 1 teaspoon onion powder
- 1 teaspoon garlic powder
- 1/8 teaspoon ground red pepper
- 1 teaspoon red chili powder
- 1 tablespoon brown sugar
- 1/4 teaspoon dry mustard powder
- 1/8 teaspoon allspice
- 1 teaspoon smoked paprika
- 1 teaspoon cumin

|Directions|

- Take a medium bowl, place all the ingredients in it, and stir well until combined.
- Transfer the rub in an air-tight glass container and store until ready to use.
- Sprinkle the rub all over the chicken piece and cook as instructed in the recipe.

Nutrition Information –

20 Cal; 4 g Carb; 0 g Protein;0 g Fat, 0 g Fiber; 9mg Sodium;34 mg Potassium; 7mg Phosphorus;

Cajun Seasoning

|Preparation Time: 5 minutes|

|Cooking Time: 0 minutes|

|Total Time: 5 minutes|

|Serve – 5 tablespoons, 2 ½ tablespoons per serving|

|Ingredients|

- 4 teaspoons onion powder
- 4 teaspoons garlic powder
- 4 teaspoons paprika
- 2 teaspoons cayenne pepper

|Directions|

- Take a medium bowl, place all the ingredients in it, and stir well until combined.
- Transfer the rub in an air-tight glass container and store until ready to use.

Nutrition Information –

25 Cal; 5 g Carb; 1 g Protein;0 g Fat, 1 g Fiber; 15mg Sodium;36mg Potassium; 5mg Phosphorus;

Chinese Five-Spice Blend

|Preparation Time: 5 minutes|

|Cooking Time: 0 minutes|

|Total Time: 5 minutes|

|Serve – ¼ cup, 1 teaspoon each serving|

|Ingredients|

- 1/2 teaspoon ground allspice mix
- 6 teaspoons ginger powder
- 1 teaspoon ground cloves
- 1 tablespoon ground cinnamon
- 1/2 teaspoon anise seed

|Directions|

- Take a medium bowl, place all the ingredients in it, and stir well until combined.
- Transfer the rub in an air-tight glass container and store until ready to use.

Nutrition Information –

20 Cal; 4 g Carb; 0 g Protein; 0 g Fat, 1 g Fiber; 14 mg Sodium; 49 mg Potassium; 4 mg Phosphorus;

Taco Seasoning

|Preparation Time: 5 minutes|

|Cooking Time: 0 minutes|

|Total Time: 5 minutes|

|Serve – ½ cup, 1 tablespoon per serving|

|Ingredients|

- 1 tablespoon onion powder
- 1 teaspoon garlic powder
- 1/4 cup red chili powder
- 1 teaspoon crushed red pepper
- 1 tablespoon ground cumin
- 1 teaspoon dried oregano
- 1/2 teaspoon cinnamon

|Directions|

- Take a medium bowl, place all the ingredients in it, and stir well until combined.
- Transfer the rub in an air-tight glass container and store until ready to use.

Nutrition Information –

14 Cal; 3 g Carb; 1 g Protein; 0 g Fat, 1 g Fiber; 3 mg Sodium; 34 mg Potassium; 9 mg Phosphorus;

Mexican Blend

|Preparation Time: 5 minutes|

|Cooking Time: 0 minutes|

|Total Time: 5 minutes|

|Serve – ½ cup, 2 tablespoons per serving|

|Ingredients|

- 1 tablespoon onion powder
- 1 teaspoon garlic powder
- 1 teaspoon crushed red pepper
- 1/4 cup red chili powder
- 1 tablespoon ground cumin
- 1 teaspoon dried oregano
- 1/2 teaspoon cinnamon

|Directions|

- Take a medium bowl, place all the ingredients in it, and stir well until combined.
- Transfer the rub in an air-tight glass container and store until ready to use.

Nutrition Information –

16 Cal; 4 g Carb; 0 g Protein; 0 g Fat, 1 g Fiber; 14 mg Sodium; 49 mg Potassium; 4 mg Phosphorus;

Mixed Herb Blend

|Preparation Time: 5 minutes|

|Cooking Time: 0 minutes|

|Total Time: 5 minutes|

|Serve – 1/3 cup, 2 tablespoons per serving|

|Ingredients|

- 1 tablespoon celery seed
- 2 tablespoons dried tarragon
- 1/4 cup dried parsley
- 1 tablespoon dried oregano
- 1 tablespoon dill weed

|Directions|

- Take a medium bowl, place all the ingredients in it, and stir well until combined.
- Transfer the rub in an air-tight glass container and store until ready to use.

Nutrition Information –

20 Cal; 4 g Carb; 0 g Protein;0 g Fat, 0 g Fiber; 9mg Sodium;34 mg Potassium; 7mg Phosphorus;

Poultry Seasoning

|Preparation Time: 5 minutes|

|Cooking Time: 0 minutes|

|Total Time: 5 minutes|

|Serve – 11 teaspoons, 1 teaspoon per serving|

|Ingredients|

- 1 teaspoon ground black pepper
- 2 teaspoons dried marjoram
- 2 tablespoons dried ground sage
- 2 teaspoons dried thyme

|Directions|

- Take a medium bowl, place all the ingredients in it, and stir well until combined.
- Transfer the rub in an air-tight glass container and store until ready to use.

Nutrition Information –

3 Cal; 0 g Carb; 0 g Protein; 0 g Fat, 0 g Fiber; 0 mg Sodium; 8 mg Potassium; 1 mg Phosphorus;

Fajita Flavor Marinade

|Preparation Time: 5 minutes|

|Cooking Time: 0 minutes|

|Total Time: 5 minutes|

|Serve – 1 cup|

|Ingredients|

- 1 jalapeño pepper, finely diced
- 1 medium grapefruit, juiced
- 1/4 teaspoon garlic powder
- 2 medium limes, juiced
- 3 tablespoons olive oil
- 1 medium orange, juiced

|Directions|

- Take a medium bowl, place all the ingredients in it, and stir well until combined.
- Pour the marinade over chicken or vegetables, toss until well coated, and let marinate for 1 hour.
- Drizzle the marinade over chicken or vegetables and cook as instructed in the recipe.

Nutrition Information –

33 Cal; 2 g Carb; 0 g Protein; 2.8 g Fat, 1 g Fiber; 0 mg Sodium; 42 mg Potassium; 5 mg Phosphorus;

Garlic-Herb Seasoning

|Preparation Time: 5 minutes|

|Cooking Time: 0 minutes|

|Total Time: 5 minutes|

|Serve – 1 ½ tablespoon, 1 tablespoon per serving|

|Ingredients|

- 2 teaspoons garlic powder
- 1 teaspoon powdered lemon rind
- 1 teaspoon dried oregano
- 1 teaspoon dried basil

|Directions|

- Add all the ingredients in the order in a food processor or blender and blend at medium speed until combined.
- Tip the mixture in an air-tight glass container, add a few grains of rice to keep the mixture from clumping and store until ready to use.

Nutrition Information –

12 Cal; 3 g Carb; 0 g Protein; 0 g Fat, 1 g Fiber; 1 mg Sodium; 47 mg Potassium; 16 mg Phosphorus;

Honey Mustard

|Preparation Time: 5 minutes|

|Cooking Time: 0 minutes|

|Total Time: 5 minutes|

|Serve – 1 cup, 1 tablespoon per serving|

|Ingredients|

- ½ teaspoon onion powder
- 1 teaspoon garlic powder
- ¼ teaspoon ground white pepper
- 1 tablespoon ground mustard
- ¼ cup honey
- ¼ cup white vinegar
- ¾ cup olive oil

|Directions|

- Add all the ingredients in the order in a food processor or blender, except for oil and honey, and pulse at medium speed until blended.
- Slowly blend in oil until incorporated and then mix in honey, 1 tablespoon at a time, until mustard reaches to desired sweetness.
- Transfer the mustard into a bowl, then cover the bowl and store for up to 2 months in the refrigerator.
- Serve when desired.

Nutrition Information –

108 Cal; 4.9 g Carb; 0 g Protein; 10.2 g Fat, 0.3 g Fiber; 0.5 mg Sodium; 11.7 mg Potassium; 25 mg Phosphorus;

Soy Sauce

|Preparation Time: 10 minutes|

|Cooking Time: 10 minutes|

|Total Time: 20 minutes|

|Serve – 3 tablespoons|

|Ingredients|

- 1/8 teaspoon garlic powder
- 1/8 teaspoon ground black pepper
- 2 teaspoons molasses
- 1 teaspoon apple cider vinegar
- 1 tablespoon red wine vinegar
- 2 tablespoons beef broth, reduced-sodium
- 1 teaspoon sesame oil
- 1/4 cup water, hot

|Directions|

- Take a medium bowl, place all the ingredients in it, and stir until combined.

- Take a small saucepan, place it over medium-low heat, pour in soy sauce, and boil it until the sauce has reduced by half.
- Then let the sauce cool completely, pour it into an air-tight glass container, cover with the lid, place it in the refrigerator and store for up to a month.
- Serve when desired.

Nutrition Information –

23 Cal; 3 g Carb; 0 g Protein; 1 g Fat, 0 g Fiber; 25 mg Sodium; 27 mg Potassium; 6 mg Phosphorus;

Barbecue Sauce

|Preparation Time: 5 minutes|

|Cooking Time: 15 minutes|

|Total Time: 20 minutes|

|Serve – 1 cup, 1 tablespoon per serving|

|Ingredients|

- 6 ounces tomato paste, sodium-reduced
- 3 tablespoons water
- 1/4 cup dark molasses
- 1/2 cup sautéed onion, minced
- 1/8 cup apple cider vinegar
- 2 tablespoons brown sugar
- 1 tablespoon Worcestershire sauce

- 1 tablespoon mustard
- 1 teaspoon lemon juice
- 1 1/2 teaspoons BBQ rub for chicken

|Directions|

- Take a medium bowl, place all the ingredients in it, and stir until combined.
- Take a small saucepan, place it over low heat, pour in barbecue sauce, and cook for 15 minutes.
- Then let the sauce cool completely, pour it into an air-tight glass container, cover with the lid, and place it in the refrigerator, and store for up to two weeks.
- Serve when desired.

Nutrition Information –

34 Cal; 8 g Carb; 0 g Protein; 0 g Fat, 2 g Fiber; 53 mg Sodium; 214 mg Potassium; 2 mg Phosphorus;

Teriyaki Sauce

|Preparation Time: 5 minutes|

|Cooking Time: 10 minutes|

|Total Time: 15 minutes|

|Serve – 1 cup, 1 tablespoon per serving|

|Ingredients|

- 1 ½ teaspoon minced garlic
- 1/2 cup brown sugar
- 1/4 teaspoon ground ginger
- 2 tablespoons Chinese sweet rice wine
- 2 tablespoons sesame oil
- 1 cup soy sauce, sodium-reduced

|Directions|

- Take a small saucepan, place it over low heat, add all the ingredients in it, stir until just mixed, and cook for 5 to 10 minutes until the sugar has dissolved.
- Then let the sauce cool completely, pour it into an air-tight glass container, cover with the lid, then keep it in the refrigerator and store for up to 1 month.
- Serve when desired.

Nutrition Information –

29 Cal; 5 g Carb; 1 g Protein; 0 g Fat, 1 g Fiber; 308 mg Sodium; 1 mg Potassium; 308 mg Phosphorus;

Pizza Sauce

|Preparation Time: 10 minutes|

|Cooking Time: 20 minutes|

|Total Time: 30 minutes|

|Serve – for a 12-inch pizza|

|Ingredients|

- 6 ounces tomato paste, sodium-reduced
- 2 tablespoons fresh basil
- 1 teaspoon dried oregano
- 2 tablespoons olive oil
- 1 teaspoon dried parsley
- 3 tablespoons water

|Directions|

- Take a medium bowl, add all the ingredients in it and stir until well mixed.
- Pour the sauce into an air-tight glass container, cover with the lid, and store in the refrigerator for up to two weeks.
- For serving, spread the sauce over a 12-inch pizza crust, then scatter with topping, and bake as instructed in the recipe.

Nutrition Information –

68 Cal; 9 g Carb; 1 g Protein; 3 g Fat, 3 g Fiber; 131 mg Sodium; 409 mg Potassium; 2 mg Phosphorus;

Alfredo Sauce

|Preparation Time: 5 minutes|

|Cooking Time: 15 minutes|

|Total Time: 20 minutes|

|Serve – 1 ¾ cup|

|Ingredients|

- 3 tablespoons all-purpose flour
- ½ teaspoon minced garlic
- 1/4 teaspoon ground nutmeg
- 1/4 cup olive oil
- 1 tablespoon lemon juice
- 2 cups of rice milk, unsweetened
- 4 ounces cream cheese, sodium-reduced
- 1/3 cup grated parmesan cheese, sodium-reduced

|Directions|

- Take a large skillet, place it over medium heat, add oil in it and when hot, add flour and whisk until well mixed.
- Then stir in garlic and pour in milk, whisking continuously until smooth and bring the mixture to boil.
- Continue cooking the sauce for 5 to 10 minutes until it has thickened to desired consistency or reduced by half, then stir in cream cheese until combined and remove the pan from heat.
- Add remaining ingredients into the sauce, stir well until mixed, and let cool for 10 minutes.
- Ladle sauce over broiled rice, steamed vegetables cooked chicken, etc. and serve.

Nutrition Information –

173 Cal; 9 g Carb; 3 g Protein; 14 g Fat, 2 g Fiber; 142 mg Sodium; 32 mg Potassium; 75 mg Phosphorus;

Tomato Salsa

|Preparation Time: 5 minutes|

|Cooking Time: 0 minutes|

|Total Time: 5 minutes|

|Serve – 1 cup|

|Ingredients|

- 2green onions, chopped
- 1 medium green bell pepper, cored, chopped
- 1jalapeño pepper, chopped
- 4Roma tomatoes, chopped
- 1/2bunch fresh cilantro, chopped
- 1 ½ teaspoon minced garlic
- 1 tablespoon dried oregano
- 1/2 teaspoon cumin

|Directions|

- Add all the ingredients in the order in a blender or food processor and pulse for 2 minutes until mixed well and chunky.
- Tip the salsa in an 8-ounce pint jar, cover it and let cool for 3 hours.
- Store the salsa for up to two weeks in a refrigerator and serve with tortilla chips.

Nutrition Information –

14 Cal; 2 g Carb; 1 g Protein; 1 g Fat, 0 g Fiber; 4 mg Sodium; 117 mg Potassium; 14 mg Phosphorus;

Basil Oil

|Preparation Time: 1 hour and 10 minutes

|Cooking Time: 5 minutes|

|Total Time: 1 hour and 15 minutes|

|Serve – 1 ¼ cup|

|Ingredients|

- 1 1/2 cups basil leaves, fresh
- 1 cup olive oil

|Directions|

- Rinse the basil leaves in a colander, drain well and pat dry with paper towels.
- Transfer basil leaves in a food processor, pour in oil and pulse until basil has finely chopped, don't puree.
- Take a saucepan, place it over medium heat, pour in the basil-oil mixture, and cook for 4 to 5 minutes until oil bubbles around the sides of pan and temperature of oil reach to 165 degrees F.

- Remove the saucepan from the cooking range and let it rest at room temperature for 1 hour until cooled.
- Take a wire strainer, line it with two layers of cheesecloth, then place it over a small bowl, pour the cooled basil-oil mixture into it, and let it pass through into the bowl.
- Press the basil to extract the remaining oil and then discard the basil.
- Pour the oil into an air-tight glass container and store in the refrigerator for up to three months.
- When ready to use, let the oil rest at room temperature for 5 minutes or more until it liquefies and then serve as desired.

Nutrition Information –

135 Cal; 0 g Carb; 0 g Protein; 15 g Fat, 15 g Fiber; 0 mg Sodium; 5 mg Potassium; 0 mg Phosphorus;

Ranch Dressing

|Preparation Time: 10 minutes|

|Cooking Time: 0 minutes|

|Total Time: 10 minutes|

|Serve – 1 cup|

|Ingredients|

- 1/2 cup mayonnaise, sodium-reduced
- 1 tablespoon fresh chives, chopped
- 1/4 teaspoon garlic powder
- 1 tablespoon dried dill
- 1 tablespoon fresh oregano, chopped
- 2 tablespoons apple cider vinegar
- 1/2 cup almond milk, unsweetened

|Directions|

- Take a medium bowl, pour in milk, add mayonnaise and vinegar and whisk until combined.
- Then add remaining ingredients and whisk until well combined.
- Spoon the dressing in an air-tight glass container and place it in the refrigerator for 1 hour or until flavors are developed.
- Place the container in the refrigerator, store it for up to 1 month and stir it well before serving.

Nutrition Information –

83 Cal; 1 g Carb; 1 g Protein; 1 g Fat, 0 g Fiber; 64 mg Sodium; 9 mg Potassium; 1 mg Phosphorus;

Turkey Broth

|Preparation Time: 10 minutes|

|Cooking Time: 2 hours and 10 minutes|

|Total Time: 2 hours and 20 minutes|

|Serve – 2 cups|

|Ingredients|

- 1 small turkey, pastured
- 2 medium white onions, peeled, quartered
- 2 medium carrots, peeled, diced
- 2stalks of celery
- 1/2 teaspoon dried thyme
- 1/2 teaspoon ground black pepper
- 2bay leaves
- 16 cups water

|Directions|

- Take a large pot, place it over medium-high heat, add all the ingredients in it, stir until mixed, and bring the mixture to boil.
- Then lower the heat to medium-low level, simmer the mixture for 2 hours, skimming foam from the top and strain the broth, discarding meat, bones, and vegetables.
- Let the broth cool for 30 minutes, store the broth in the freezer and reheat it when ready to serve.

Nutrition Information –

30 Cal; 2 g Carb; 4 g Protein; 0.7 g Fat, 0.9 g Fiber; 70 mg Sodium; 200 mg Potassium; 70 mg Phosphorus;

Pickles

|Preparation Time: 10 minutes|

|Cooking Time: 0 minutes|

|Total Time: 10 minutes|

|Serve – 58 servings|

|Ingredients|

- 5English cucumbers, sliced
- 1 teaspoon ground black pepper
- 2 cups brown sugar
- 1/2 teaspoon dry mustard
- 1 teaspoon ground turmeric
- 1 1/2 cups red wine vinegar
- 2 teaspoons celery seed
- 2 tablespoons dill weed
- 1 1/2 cups apple cider vinegar
- 1 bunch fresh dill
- 2 cups white wine vinegar

|Directions|

- Prepare the cucumbers - slice them, then layer them evenly in pint jars and evenly fill the jars

with black pepper, mustard, turmeric, celery, dill weed, and dill.
- Pour all the kinds of vinegar in a pitcher, add brown sugar, and stir well until sugar has dissolved.
- Pour the vinegar mixture into pint jars, leaving some space at the top, and then cover the jars with lids.
- Place the jars in the refrigerator and store them for up to six months.

Nutrition Information –

30 Cal; 7 g Carb; 0 g Protein; 0 g Fat, 2.5 g Fiber; 1 mg Sodium; 15 mg Potassium; 2 mg Phosphorus;

Part 5 – Meal Planning For Renal Diet

30-Day Meal Plan

Week 1

Day 1

Breakfast: Egg and Sausage Breakfast Sandwich

Lunch: Seafood Corn Chowder

Dinner: Vegetarian Egg Fried Rice

Dessert: Crepes with Frozen Berries

Day 2

Breakfast: Strawberry and Cream Cheese French Toast Casserole

Lunch: Vegetarian Pizza

Dinner: Creamy Shells with Peas and Bacon

Dessert: Crepes with Frozen Berries

Day 3

Breakfast: "Berrylicious" Smoothie

Lunch: Chicken Noodle Soup

Dinner: Salmon Burgers with Coleslaw

Dessert: Low Phosphorus Fudge

Day 4

Breakfast: Zucchini Pancakes

Lunch: Eggplant Seafood Casserole

Dinner: Cauliflower and Broccoli Mac-n-Cheese

Dessert: Low Phosphorus Fudge

Day 5

Breakfast: Southern-style Cornbread

Lunch: Korean-Style Fried Fish

Dinner: Pita Pizza

Dessert: Cranberry and Apple Salad

Day 6

Breakfast: Vegetables Omelet

Lunch: Lemon Rice with Vegetables

Dinner: Cauliflower Manchurian

Dessert: Banana Dessert

Day 7

Breakfast: Asparagus and Cauliflower Tortilla

Lunch: Veggie Strata

Dinner: Feta Pasta with Chicken and Asparagus

Dessert: Banana Dessert

Week 2

Day 8

Breakfast: Cranberry and Roasted Garlic Risotto

Lunch: Flavorful Grilled Salmon

Dinner: Tuna Noodle Casserole

Dessert: Stuffed Strawberries

Day 9

Breakfast: Old Fashion Waffles

Lunch: Chiles Rellenos

Dinner: Ratatouille

Dessert: Stuffed Strawberries

Day 10

Breakfast: Lemon Apple Honey Smoothie

Lunch: Pumpkin Chili

Dinner: Chicken Wild Rice Soup

Dessert: Sugarless Heart Cookies

Day 11

Breakfast: Cheese Pancakes with Strawberries

Lunch: Buffalo Wings

Dinner: Broiled Haddock with Cucumber Salsa

Dessert: Sugarless Heart Cookies

Day 12

Breakfast: Potato Gratin

Lunch: Crab Cakes

Dinner: Tofu Stir Fry

Dessert: Pear Crisp

Day 13

Breakfast: Breakfast Burrito

Lunch: Deviled Green Beans

Dinner: Chicken Parmesan Meatballs

Dessert: Berry Galette

Day 14

Breakfast: Wheat and Berry Breakfast Bowl

Lunch: Triple Berry Salad

Dinner: Mediterranean Pizza

Dessert: Berry Galette

Week 3

Day 15

Breakfast: Omelet

Lunch: Salmon and Summer Squash

Dinner: Chicken Lettuce Wraps

Dessert: Cherry Coffee Cake

Day 16

Breakfast: Banana Oat Shake

Lunch: Cranberry Cabbage

Dinner: Salmon Steaks with Herb Dressing

Dessert: Cherry Coffee Cake

Day 17

Breakfast: Gingersnap Cookies

Lunch: Potato Salad

Dinner: Creamy Orzo and Vegetables

Dessert: Cherry Coffee Cake

Day 18

Breakfast: Corn Cakes with Cheese

Lunch: Tortilla Pizza

Dinner: Honey Mustard Grilled Chicken

Dessert: Creamy Grape Salad

Day 19

Breakfast: Zucchini Frittata

Lunch: Shrimp Fried Rice

Dinner: Roasted Brussels Sprouts, Carrots and Apples

Dessert: Caramel Custard

Day 20

Breakfast: Bagel with Egg and Salmon

Lunch: Mashed Cauliflower Potatoes

Dinner: Citrus Salmon

Dessert: Caramel Custard

Day 21

Breakfast: Banana and Apple Smoothie

Lunch: Pasta Primavera

Dinner: Italian Style Vegetables & Pasta with Chicken

Dessert: Dessert Pizza

Week 4

Day 22

Breakfast: Fruity Dump Cake

Lunch: Tempeh Pita Sandwiches

Dinner: Vegetable Casserole Delite

Dessert:Dessert Pizza

Day 23

Breakfast: Cottage Cheese and Sour Cream Pancakes

Lunch: Shrimp and Broccoli Fettuccine

Dinner: Chicken Chili

Dessert: Berries Napoleon

Day 24

Breakfast: Fruit Lassi

Lunch: Singapore Rice Noodles

Dinner: Penne Pasta with Asparagus

Dessert: Berries Napoleon

Day 25

Breakfast: Short Bread Cookies

Lunch: Gratin Pasta with Chicken and Watercress

Dinner: Salmon Soup

Dessert: Carrot Cake

Day 26

Breakfast: Apple and Onion Omelet

Lunch: Cranberry Rice Pilaf

Dinner: Macaroni and Cheese

Dessert: Carrot Cake

Day 27

Breakfast: Stuffed French Toast

Lunch: Grilled Salmon Sandwiches

Dinner: Glazed Cornish Game Hen

Dessert: Orange Pineapple Ambrosia Salad

Day 28

Breakfast: Berry Smoothie Bowl

Lunch: Buffalo Chicken Dip

Dinner: Honey Spice-Rubbed Salmon

Dessert: Low Phosphorus Fudge

Week 5

Day 29

Breakfast: Spaghetti-Basil Frittata

Lunch: Autumn Wild Rice

Dinner: Mexican Chicken Pizza

Dessert: Sugarless Heart Cookies

Day 30

Breakfast: Clam Omelet

Lunch: Fish Fry with Seasoned Rice

Dinner: Hawaiian Rice

Dessert: Sugarless Heart Cookies

Week 1 Shopping List

Meat, Poultry and Meat Substitutes

- Tofu, extra-firm – 1 cup
- Tofu, silken – 1 1/3 cup
- Chicken – 16 ounce
- Chicken broth – 3 ½ cups
- Turkey sausage patty - 1
- Slices of bacon – 3
- Pork, ground – 2 ounces

Fish and Seafood

- Crabmeat – 1 ½ pound
- Salmon – 15 ounces
- Shrimps – ½ pound
- Whitefish fillets – 1 pound

Vegetables

- Minced garlic – 5 ½ teaspoon
- Grated ginger – 2 tablespoons
- White onion – 15 medium
- Green onion – 3 medium
- Red onion – 1 medium
- Mushrooms, sliced – 2 cups
- Cauliflower florets – 6 cups
- Broccoli florets – 2 cups

- Carrot – 3 medium
- Celery – 3
- Spinach – 15 leaves
- Asparagus – 2 pounds
- Green bell pepper – 4 medium
- Red bell pepper – 3 medium
- Green peas – 1 1/4 cup
- Cilantro – ½ bunch
- Lemon juice – ½ cup
- Coleslaw mix – 5 cups
- Zucchini – 5 medium
- Eggplant – 2 medium

Fruits

- Mixed berries, frozen – ½ cup
- Fresh strawberries – 2 cups
- Frozen raspberries – 1 cup
- Frozen blueberries – 1 cup
- Pineapple chunks – 1/2 cup
- Apple – 4 medium

Breads, Cereals, and Pasta

- Breadcrumbs – 2 cup
- All-purpose white flour – 4 cup
- Corn kernels – 2 ¼ cups
- Cornmeal – 2 cups
- Long grain rice – 5 cups

- Rice flour – 2 tablespoons
- Rice drink – 2 ½ cups
- Whole wheat shell pasta – 1 ½ cup
- Egg noodles – 2 ounce
- Penne pasta – 28 ounce
- Pita bread – 2

Dairy and Dairy Alternatives

- Eggs – 29
- Liquid egg substitute – 1 1/2 cup
- Cheddar cheese, shredded – 1 1/3 cup
- Mozzarella cheese, shredded – 2/3 cup
- Parmesan cheese, grated – 1 cup
- Swiss cheese, shredded – 1 cup
- Feta cheese, crumbled – ¼ cup
- Half-and-half creamer – 6 cups
- Creamer, nondairy – ½ cup
- Cream cheese – 12 ounces
- Evaporated milk, unsweetened – 6 ounces
- Almond milk – ½ cup
- Rice milk – 2 ½ cups
- Yogurt – 1 cup

Spices and Herbs

- Chopped parsley – 2 tablespoons
- Salt – 1 1/3 teaspoon
- White sugar – 2 ¼ cup

- Powdered sugar – 1 tablespoon
- Coconut Sugar – 3/4 cup
- Maple syrup – 1/3 cup
- Splenda – ¼ cup
- Fruit protector – 1 tablespoon
- Red chili powder – 1/2 teaspoon
- Curry powder – 1 teaspoon
- Cumin powder – 1/2 teaspoon
- Paprika – 1/2 teaspoon
- Black pepper – 3 ½ teaspoon
- Poultry seasoning – ¼ teaspoon
- Dry mustard – 3 tablespoons
- Cayenne pepper – 1/8 teaspoon
- Red pepper flakes – ¼ teaspoon
- Creole seasoning – ¼ teaspoon
- Nutmeg – 1/2 teaspoon
- Onion powder – 1/8 teaspoon
- Garlic powder – 1/3 teaspoon
- Garlic and herb seasoning blend – 2 teaspoons
- Dried dill – 1/4 teaspoon
- Dried thyme – 1/2 teaspoon
- Fennel seeds – ½ teaspoon
- Lemon zest – 1 teaspoon
- Yeast – 1 envelope
- Worcestershire sauce – 2 tablespoons

- Tabasco sauce – 1 ½ teaspoon
- Soy sauce – 2 tablespoon
- White vinegar – 3 tablespoon
- Rice vinegar, unseasoned – 1 tablespoon
- Tarragon vinegar – 1/4 cup
- Powdered lemonade – 1 teaspoon
- Vanilla extract – 3 teaspoon
- Chocolate chips – 1 ½ cups

Fat and Oil

- Canola oil – 4 1/3 cups
- Olive oil – 1 cup
- Sesame oil – ¼ cup
- Unsalted butter – 1 cup
- Unsalted margarine – 1 tablespoon

Other

- English muffin – 1
- Sourdough bread – 2
- Pizza dough – 1
- Roasted red pepper tomato sauce – 1 cup
- Tomato sauce – 2 tablespoons
- Cranberry juice cocktail – ½ cup
- Marshmallows – 2 ½ cups
- Banana cream pudding mix – 7 ounce
- Vanilla wafers – 12 ounce

Week 2 Shopping List

Meat, Poultry and Meat Substitutes

- Ground turkey – 2 pounds
- Tofu, extra-firm – 16 ounces
- Chicken – 8 ounces
- Ground chicken – 1 pound
- Chicken wings – 24
- Chicken broth – 10 cups

Fish and Seafood

- Crabmeat – 1 pound
- Salmon – 24 ounces
- Haddock – 1 pound
- Tuna, packed in water – 5 ounces

Vegetables

- Garlic cloves – 4
- Minced garlic – 5 ½ teaspoons
- Crystallized ginger – 2 tablespoons
- White onion – 6
- White potato – 1 ¼ pound
- Tomato – 2 medium
- Roma tomato 1
- Green beans 2 cups
- Red onion – 1 medium

- Mushrooms, sliced – 1 cup
- Broccoli florets – 1 cup
- Carrot – 6
- Green chilies – 9
- Green chili pepper – 2
- Cucumber 1
- Celery – 2
- Green bell pepper – 2
- Red bell pepper – 5 ½ medium
- Yellow bell pepper – 1 medium
- Yellow crookneck squash – 3
- Green peas – ½ cup
- Cilantro – 3 tablespoons
- Capers – 1 tablespoon
- Lemon – 2
- Lemon juice – 1 cup
- Lime juice – 6 tablespoons
- Zucchini – 2
- Eggplant – 1

Fruits

- dried cranberries – 1/2 cup
- Fresh cranberries – ½ cup
- Wheat berries – ½ cup
- Banana – 1
- Pears – 3 pounds

- Mixed berries, frozen – 2 cups
- Fresh strawberries, whole – 24
- Fresh strawberries, sliced – 5 cups
- Pear – 1 medium
- Frozen blueberries – 1 cup
- Fresh blackberries – 1 cup
- Apple – 1
- Apple juice – ½ cup
- Pumpkin puree – 15 ounces
- Lemon – 1

Breads, Beans, Cereals, and Pasta

- Breadcrumbs – 1 cup
- All-purpose white flour – 5 ¼ cup
- Red kidney beans – 1 cup
- Long grain rice – 2 cups
- Arborio rice – 3/4 cup
- Wild rice and long grain rice blend – 2/3 cup
- Egg noodles – 2 ounces
- Flour tortilla – 2
- Pie crust – 1
- Pizza crust – 1

Dairy and Dairy Alternatives

- Eggs – 15
- Liquid egg substitute – ¼ cup

- Mozzarella cheese, shredded – ½ cup
- Parmesan cheese, grated – 1 ½ cup
- Goat cheese – 3 ounces
- Cottage cheese – 3 ¼ cup
- Cream cheese – 1 cup
- Sour cream – ¾ cup
- Almond milk – 2 ¾ cup
- Yogurt – 1 cup

Spices and Herbs

- Almonds – 1 tablespoon
- Walnuts – ¾ cup
- Sesame seeds – ½ teaspoon
- Chopped parsley – 2 tablespoons
- Salt – 1 teaspoon
- White sugar – 2 teaspoons
- Brown sugar – ¼ cup
- Coconut sugar – ½ cup
- Maple syrup – 2 tablespoons
- Honey – 2 teaspoons
- Blackberry preserves – 1 tablespoon
- Mixed fruit gelatin – 1 small box
- Baking powder – ½ teaspoon
- Red chili powder – 1 tablespoon
- Cinnamon – 1 teaspoon
- Cumin powder – 2 ¼ teaspoons

- Black pepper – 2 tablespoons
- Dry mustard – 3 tablespoons
- Cornstarch – 3 tablespoons
- Mayonnaise – ¼ cup
- Cayenne pepper – 1/8 teaspoon
- Nutmeg – 1/8 teaspoon
- Onion powder – ¾ teaspoon
- Minced onion – 1 tablespoon
- Garlic powder –3 tablespoons
- Garlic and herb seasoning blend – 1½ teaspoon
- Italian seasoning blend – 3/4 teaspoon
- Cayenne pepper – 1/3 teaspoon
- Fresh thyme – 1 tablespoon
- Fresh sage 1 tablespoon
- Fresh basil, chopped – 1 tablespoon
- Fresh basil – 10 leaves
- Fresh oregano – 1 tablespoon
- Dried oregano – 1 teaspoon
- Fresh rosemary – 2 tablespoons
- Orange zest – 1 teaspoon
- Bay leaves – 2
- Yeast – 1 ½ teaspoon
- White wine – ¾ cup
- Worcestershire sauce – 1 teaspoon
- Tabasco sauce – 1/3 cup

- Soy sauce – 1 ½ tablespoon
- Hot pepper sauce – ½ teaspoon
- Vanilla extract – 1 teaspoon
- Almond extract – 1 teaspoon

Fat and Oil

- Canola oil – 1 1/8 cup
- Olive oil – ¾ cup
- Sesame oil – 1 tablespoon
- Unsalted butter – 2 ½ cup
- Unsalted margarine – 1 ¼ cup

Other

- Crushed cracker – 6
- Red pepper sauce – ¼ cup
- Pizza sauce – 8 ounces
- Tomato sauce – ¼ cup

Week 3 Shopping List

Meat, Poultry and Meat Substitutes

- Chicken – 2 pounds
- Chicken broth – 6 cups

Fish and Seafood

- Salmon – 4 pound
- Shrimps, small – ½ cup

Vegetables

- Minced garlic – 5 teaspoons
- Ground ginger – 1 tablespoon
- Grated ginger – 2 tablespoons
- Candied ginger – ½ cup
- White onion – 6
- Shallot – 1 small
- White potato – 3 medium
- Red potato 1 medium
- Tomato – 1 small
- Green onion – 2
- Scallion – 3
- Red onion – 1 medium
- Mushrooms, sliced – ½ cup
- Cauliflower florets – 8 ounces
- Broccoli florets – ¾ cup

- Carrot – 6 medium
- Brussels sprouts – 20 medium
- Celery – 2 medium
- Green bell pepper – 3 medium
- Red bell pepper – 2 medium
- Yellow crookneck squash – 2
- Green peas – 1
- Cilantro, chopped – ¼ cup
- Capers – 1 tablespoon
- Lemon – 2
- Lemon juice – 1/3 cup
- Zucchini – 7 medium
- Lettuce leaves – 8
- Red cabbage – 1 medium
- Arugula – 4 pieces
- Mix vegetables – 12 ounces

Fruits

- Grapes – 3 pounds
- Banana – 3
- Fresh strawberries, sliced – 1 cup
- Peaches, sliced – 1 cup
- Apple – 6

Breads, Beans, Cereals, and Pasta

- Oatmeal – 1 cup
- Oat bran – ½ cup

- What germ – 2 tablespoons
- All-purpose white flour – 4 cups 2 tablespoons
- Long grain rice – 4 cups
- Wild rice – ½ cup
- Converted rice – ¾ cup
- Penne pasta – 12 ounces
- Orzo pasta – 1 cup
- Pasta twists – 1 cup
- Flour tortilla – 2
- Pizza crust – 1
- Bagel – 1/2

Dairy and Dairy Alternatives

- Eggs – 21
- Parmesan cheese, grated – 1 cup
- Costeño cheese, grated – 4 ounces
- Half-and-half creamer – ¼ cup
- Cream cheese – 12 ounces
- Sour cream – 2 cups
- Almond milk – 2 1/3 cup
- Buttermilk – 3 tablespoons
- Coconut milk – 3 cups
- Yogurt – 2 cups

Spices and Herbs

- Chopped parsley – ½ cup

- Dried parsley – 1 teaspoon
- Salt – 1/3 teaspoon
- White sugar – 1 ¼ cup
- Brown sugar – 2 cups 4 tablespoons
- Dark molasses – ¼ cup
- Cinnamon sugar – ½ cup
- Powdered sugar – 1/3 cup
- Maple syrup – 2 tablespoons
- Honey – 5 tablespoons
- Ground cloves – ¼ teaspoon
- Chinese Five Spice Seasoning – 1 teaspoon
- Baking soda – 3 teaspoons
- Baking powder – 1 teaspoon
- Anise – ½ teaspoon
- Cinnamon – 1 teaspoon
- Curry powder – 1 teaspoon
- Black pepper – 2 teaspoons
- Black peppercorns – 10
- Dried marjoram – ½ teaspoon
- Dry mustard – 3 tablespoons
- White corn flour – 2/3 cup
- Cornstarch – 2 teaspoons
- Mayonnaise – 2 cups
- Cayenne pepper – ¼ teaspoon
- Red pepper flakes – ¼ teaspoon
- Nutmeg – ½ teaspoon

- Garlic powder – 1 teaspoon
- Dried dill – 1 teaspoon
- Fresh dill – ½ teaspoon
- Dill weed – 1/3 cup
- Fresh chives – 1 tablespoon
- Fresh sage sprig – 1
- Fresh basil leaves – 4
- Dried basil – 1 teaspoon
- Dried rosemary – 1 teaspoon
- Bay leaves – 2
- Hoisin sauce – 2 teaspoons
- Apple cider vinegar – ¼ cup
- Red wine vinegar – 2 tablespoons
- Rice vinegar, unseasoned – 2 tablespoons
- Vanilla extract – 3 tablespoons
- Chocolate chips – ¼ cup

Fat and Oil

- Canola oil – 2/3 cup
- Olive oil – 1 cup
- Sesame oil – 2 tablespoons
- Peanut oil – 5 tablespoons
- Unsalted butter –1 ½ cup
- Unsalted margarine – 2 tablespoons

Other

- Baking mix – 1 cup

- Cherry pie filling – 20 ounces
- Whole-berry cranberry sauce – 10 ounces
- Warm jelly – 2 tablespoons
- Applesauce – 2 cups
- Apricot jam – ½ cup
- Marinara sauce – 4 tablespoons

Week 4 Shopping List

Meat, Poultry and Meat Substitutes

- Chicken – 3 pounds
- Cornish game hen – 1 ¼ pound
- Chicken broth – 2 cups 28 ounces
- Tempeh – 8 ounces

Fish and Seafood

- Salmon – 3 pound
- Shrimps, small – ¾ pound

Vegetables

- Minced garlic – ½ cup
- White onion – 6 small
- Sweet onion – 2
- Watercress, chopped – 1 cup
- Roasted red peppers – 8
- Tomato – 2 medium
- Scallion – 4
- Green beans – ½ cup
- Mushrooms, sliced – 1/2 cup
- Broccoli florets – 2 cups
- Carrot – 17 medium
- Snow peas, sliced – 1 cup
- Green chilies – 4 ounces
- Celery – 5

- Asparagus – 1 pound
- Green bell pepper – 2
- Red bell pepper – 2
- Yellow summer squash – 1
- Cilantro – ½ bunch
- Lemon juice – ¼ cup 2 teaspoons
- Lime juice – ½ cup 1 tablespoon
- Arugula – 4 cups

Fruits

- Dried cranberries – 2 tablespoons
- Maraschino cherries – 8
- Orange – 11 ounces
- Mixed berries, frozen – 2 tablespoons
- Peaches, sliced – 40 ounces
- Frozen raspberries – ½ cup
- Frozen blueberries – 1 cup
- Mango juice – 1 cup
- Pineapple, crushed – 8 ounces
- Apple – 1 large
- Frozen acai – 1 packet

Breads, Beans, Cereals, and Pasta

- All-purpose white flour – 2 ½ cup
- Red kidney beans – 1 cup
- Long grain rice – 5 cups
- Cake flour – 2 ¼ cups

- Rice noodles – 8 ounces
- Penne pasta – 8 ounces
- Fettucine pasta 4 ounces
- Elbow pasta – 1 cup
- Pasta shells – 2 cups
- Pita bread – 2

Dairy and Dairy Alternatives

- Eggs – 11
- Liquid egg whites – 8 ounces
- Liquid egg substitute – ¼ cup
- Whipped topping – 1 cup
- Cheddar cheese, shredded – ½ cup 2 tablespoons
- Parmesan cheese, grated – 3/4 cup
- Pimento Cheese spread made with cream cheese – 5 ounces
- Cottage cheese – ½ cup
- Half-and-half creamer – 12 ounces
- Cream cheese – 23 ounces
- Sour cream – 2 cups
- Almond milk – 1 ¼ cup
- Coconut milk – 2 cups
- Yogurt – 2 cups

Spices and Herbs

- Chia seeds – 1 teaspoon
- Salt – 2/3 teaspoon

- White sugar – 1 2/3 cups
- Brown sugar – 1 ¼ cup
- Swerve sugar 1 tablespoon
- Splenda – 1 ¾ cup
- Cinnamon stick – 1
- Cardamom – ½ teaspoon
- Black cumin – ½ teaspoon
- Honey – 3 tablespoons
- Baking soda – ½ teaspoon
- Baking powder – 1 teaspoon
- Red chili powder – 3 tablespoons
- Cinnamon – 2 tablespoons
- Curry powder – 1 tablespoon
- Paprika – 1/8 teaspoon
- Black pepper – 2 ½ teaspoons
- Black peppercorns, ground – ¾ teaspoon
- Dry mustard – 1 teaspoon
- Cornstarch – ¼ cup
- Mayonnaise – 4 teaspoons
- Chipotle mayonnaise – ¼ cup
- Red pepper flakes – 1/8 teaspoon
- Garlic powder – 2 ½ teaspoons
- Lemon-pepper seasoning ½ teaspoon
- Fresh dill sprig – 1
- Dried oregano – 1 teaspoon
- Lemon peel – ¾ teaspoon

- Bay leaf – 1
- Worcestershire sauce – 1 teaspoon
- Tabasco sauce – 5 teaspoons
- Soy sauce – 1 tablespoon
- Balsamic vinegar – 2 tablespoons
- Vanilla extract – 2 teaspoons
- Coconut, grated – 2 tablespoons
- Chocolate chips – 1 ½ cups

Fat and Oil

- Canola oil – 2 cups
- Olive oil – ½ cup
- Sesame oil – 2 tablespoons
- Unsalted butter – 3 cups

Other

- Yellowcake mix – 15.25 ounce
- Tomato salsa – ¾ cup
- Wonton wrappers – 12
- Béchamel sauce – 1 2/3 cup
- Rosewater – 1 teaspoon
- Applesauce – 2 tablespoons
- Apricot jam – 2 tablespoons
- Whole-wheat bread – 1
- Sourdough bread – 1
- Marshmallows – 2 cups

Part 6 – Recipes

Breakfast

Lemon Apple Honey Smoothie

|Preparation Time: 5 minutes|

|Cooking Time: 0 minutes|

|Total Time: 5 minutes|

|Serve – 4|

|Ingredients|

- 1 medium banana, peeled
- 1 medium apple, peeled, cored
- 2 teaspoons honey
- 1/4 cup fresh lemon juice
- 1/2 cup fresh apple juice
- 1 cup Greek yogurt

|Directions|

- Take a food processor or blender, add all the ingredients for smoothie and pulse for 1 to 2 minutes until blended and smooth.
- Divide the smoothie evenly between four chilled glasses and serve.

Nutrition Information –

170 Cal; 38 g Carb; 2 g Protein; 0g Fat, 2 g Fiber; 37 mg Sodium; 327 mg Potassium; 59 mg Phosphorus;

Banana Oat Shake

|Preparation Time: 5 minutes|

|Cooking Time: 0 minutes|

|Total Time: 5 minutes|

|Serve – 4|

|Ingredients|

- 1 frozen banana, cut into chunks
- 1 cup cooked oatmeal, chilled
- 2 tablespoons wheat germ
- 4 tablespoons brown sugar
- 3 teaspoons vanilla extract, unsweetened
- 1 1/3 cup almond milk, unsweetened

|Directions|

- Add oatmeal in a food processor or blender and pulse for 2 minutes until blended.
- Then add remaining ingredients and continue blending until smooth.
- Divide the smoothie evenly between four chilled glasses and serve.

Nutrition Information –

172 Cal; 33 g Carb; 6 g Protein; 0 g Fat, 2 g Fiber; 42 mg Sodium; 297 mg Potassium; 160 mg Phosphorus;

Banana and Apple Smoothie

|Preparation Time: 5 minutes|

|Cooking Time: 0 minutes|

|Total Time: 5 minutes|

|Serve – 4|

|Ingredients|

- ½ cup oat bran
- 2 bananas, peeled, diced
- 4 tablespoon honey
- 1 cup almond milk
- 2 cups applesauce, unsweetened
- 2 cups Greek yogurt

|Directions|

- Take a food processor or blender, add all the ingredients for smoothie in it, except for oat bran, and pulse for 1 to 2 minutes until blended.
- Then add oat bran and continue blending until smooth and thick.
- Divide the smoothie evenly between four chilled glasses and serve.

Nutrition Information –

292 Cal; 61 g Carb; 9 g Protein; 0 g Fat, 5 g Fiber; 163 mg Sodium; 609 mg Potassium; 140 mg Phosphorus;

"Berrylicious" Smoothie

|Preparation Time: 5 minutes|

|Cooking Time: 0 minutes|

|Total Time: 5 minutes|

|Serve – 4|

|Ingredients|

- 1 cup frozen raspberries, unsweetened
- 1 1/3 cup silken tofu, firm
- 1 cup frozen blueberries, unsweetened
- 1 teaspoon powdered lemonade
- 2 teaspoons vanilla extract, unsweetened
- ½ cup cranberry juice cocktail

|Directions|

- Take a food processor or blender, add all the ingredients for smoothie in it and pulse for 1 to 2 minutes until blended and smooth.
- Divide the smoothie evenly between four chilled glasses and serve.

Nutrition Information –

115 Cal; 18 g Carb; 6 g Protein; 3 g Fat, 1 g Fiber; 14 mg Sodium; 223 mg Potassium; 80 mg Phosphorus;

Fruit Lassi

|Preparation Time: 5 minutes|

|Cooking Time: 0 minutes|

|Total Time: 5 minutes|

|Serve – 4|

|Ingredients|

- 1cup fresh mango juice
- 6 tablespoons brown sugar
- 1/2 teaspoon cardamom
- 1 teaspoon rose water
- 1/2 cup lime juice
- 2 cups Greek yogurt
- 1 cup almond milk

|Directions|

- Take a food processor or blender, add all the ingredients for lassi in it and pulse for 1 to 2 minutes until blended and smooth.
- Divide the smoothie evenly between four chilled glasses and serve.

Nutrition Information –

169 Cal; 29 g Carb; 9 g Protein; 0 g Fat, 2 g Fiber; 143 mg Sodium; 98 mg Potassium; 59 mg Phosphorus;

Gingersnap Cookies

|Preparation Time: 10 minutes|

|Cooking Time: 10 minutes|

|Total Time: 20 minutes|

|Serve – 3 dozens|

|Ingredients|

- 2 cups white all-purpose white flour, low-sodium
- 1 tablespoon ground ginger
- 2 teaspoons fresh grated ginger
- 1/2 cup candied ginger, chopped
- 1 teaspoon ground cinnamon
- 1 cup brown sugar
- 1/3 cup cinnamon sugar
- 2 teaspoons baking soda
- 1/4 cup dark molasses
- 3/4 cup unsalted butter
- 1 egg

|Directions|

- Switch on the oven, then set it to 350 degrees F and let it preheat.
- Meanwhile, take a large bowl, place flour in it, add cinnamon, ginger, and baking soda and stir until mixed.

- Add butter, whisk until incorporated, then beat in brown sugar, molasses, and egg until smooth and creamy.
- Stir in flour, 1/3 cup at a time, until a soft dough comes together, stir in candied ginger and shape the dough into 1-inch diameter dough balls.
- Roll each dough ball in cinnamon sugar, arrange them on an ungreased baking sheet, and bake for 10 minutes until cookies have slightly cracked and golden brown.
- When done, transfer cookies onto a wire rack, let them cool completely and serve.

Nutrition Information –

92 Cal; 14 g Carb; 1 g Protein; 3 g Fat, 4 g Fiber; 117 mg Sodium; 57 mg Potassium; 11 mg Phosphorus;

Omelet

|Preparation Time: 5 minutes|

|Cooking Time: 5 minutes|

|Total Time: 15 minutes|

|Serve – 4|

|Ingredients|

- 1/2 cup mixed bell peppers, chopped
- 1 tablespoon unsalted butter

- 2 pasteurized eggs
- 2 tablespoons water

|Directions|

- Crack eggs in a bowl, add water and whisk until blended.
- Take a frying pan, place it over medium heat, add butter and when it starts to melt, pour in the egg mixture and cook the egg by tilting the pan, then push the uncooked egg to the edges and the cooked portion towards the center, and continue cooking until the eggs are set.
- Then top one half of the omelet with mixed vegetables and cover the filling with another half of the omelet.
- Slide omelet to a plate and serve.

Nutrition Information –

255 Cal; 4 g Carb; 13 g Protein; 15 g Fat, 2 g Fiber; 145 mg Sodium; 122 mg Potassium; 195 mg Phosphorus;

Southern-style Cornbread

|Preparation Time: 55 minutes|

|Cooking Time: 30 minutes|

|Total Time: 1 hour and 25 minutes|

|Serve – 6|

|Ingredients|

- 13/4 cup all-purpose white cornmeal
- 1 teaspoon salt
- 1 envelope of rising yeast
- 3 cups all-purpose white flour
- 1/4 cup Splenda
- 4 tablespoons unsalted butter, melted
- 1 tablespoon olive oil
- 1/2 cup creamer, nondairy
- 2 pasteurized eggs
- 1 cup of water

|Directions|

- Place 1 cup flour in a bowl, add cornmeal, yeast, salt, and sugar, and stir until mixed.
- Add creamer in another bowl, add water, whisk well and heat to 130 degrees F, and then whisk in melted butter until combined.
- Use an electric mixer to beat in flour mixture, about 3 tablespoons at a time, until incorporated and then beat in eggs at high speed until combined and stiff batter comes together.
- Place a skillet pan, grease it with oil and place it over medium-low heat until warmed.
- Remove warmed pan from heat, spoon in prepared batter, spread it evenly, then brush oil on top, cover the dough with a kitchen towel and place it in a warm place for 45 minutes or until raised.

- Meanwhile, switch on the oven, then set it to 375 degrees F and let it preheat.
- After 45 minutes, transfer the skillet pan into the oven and bake for 30 minutes until the top is golden brown and bread has firm.
- When done, let the bread cool for 10 minutes, then cut it into slices and serve.

Nutrition Information –

185 Cal; 30 g Carb; 4 g Protein; 5 g Fat, 1.6 g Fiber; 141 mg Sodium; 62 mg Potassium; 62 mg Phosphorus;

Breakfast Burrito

|Preparation Time: 10 minutes|

|Cooking Time: 5 minutes|

|Total Time: 15 minutes|

|Serve – 2|

|Ingredients|

- 2 flour tortillas, low-sodium
- 3 tablespoons green chilis, diced
- 1/4 teaspoon ground cumin
- 1/2 teaspoon hot pepper sauce
- 4 pasteurized eggs

|Directions|

- Crack eggs in a bowl, add green chilies, hot sauce and cumin and whisk until combined.
- Take a skillet pan, place it over medium heat, grease it with oil and when hot, pour in eggs and cook for 2 minutes until done.
- Prepare burritos, and for this, heat them in a microwave until warm through, then place half of the cooked eggs on each tortilla and roll them up.
- Serve straight away.

Nutrition Information –

366 Cal; 33 g Carb; 18 g Protein; 18 g Fat, 2.5 g Fiber; 594 mg Sodium; 245 mg Potassium; 300 mg Phosphorus;

Vegetables Omelet

|Preparation Time: 10 minutes|

|Cooking Time: 10 minutes|

|Total Time: 20 minutes|

|Serve – 1|

|Ingredients|

- 1/4 cup frozen kernel corn, thawed
- 3 tablespoons chopped green onion
- 1/3 cup chopped zucchini
- 1/4 teaspoon garlic and herb blend

- 1 egg
- 2 egg whites
- ¼ cup shredded cheddar cheese, low-fat
- 2 tablespoons water

|Directions|

- Take a small saucepan, place it over medium-high heat, grease it with oil and when hot, add onion, zucchini, and corn and cook for 4 minutes until vegetables are tender-crisp, set aside until required.
- Crack the egg in a bowl, add egg whites, herb blend, and water and whisk until combined.
- Take a skillet pan, place it over medium-high heat, grease it with oil and when hot, add egg mixture and cook for 2 minutes until edges have set.
- Then spread the vegetables on top of half omelet, sprinkle with cheese and cover the filling with the other half.
- Continue cooking the omelet for 2 minutes or until cheese has melted and then slide omelet onto a plate.
- Serve straight away.

Nutrition Information –

187 Cal; 12 g Carb; 22 g Protein; 6 g Fat, 2.2 g Fiber; 270 mg Sodium; 352 mg Potassium; 218 mg Phosphorus;

Fruity Dump Cake

|Preparation Time: 10 minutes|

|Cooking Time: 30 minutes|

|Total Time: 40 minutes|

|Serve – 12|

|Ingredients|

- 15.25 ounces dry yellow cake mix
- 40 ounces sliced peaches
- 1/2 cup unsalted butter

|Directions|

- Switch on the oven, then set it to 350 degrees F and let it preheat.
- Meanwhile, take a heatproof bake pan, about 9 by 13 inches grease it with oil, then spread peaches evenly in it and top with cake mix.
- Dot the cake mix layer with butter and bake for 30 minutes until the top has golden brown.
- Serve straight away.

Nutrition Information –

260 Cal; 44 g Carb; 1 g Protein; 9 g Fat, 0.7 g Fiber; 292 mg Sodium; 107 mg Potassium; 140 mg Phosphorus;

Short Bread Cookies

|Preparation Time: 10 minutes|

|Cooking Time: 10 minutes|

|Total Time: 20 minutes|

|Serve – 24 cookies|

|Ingredients|

- 1 cup unsalted butter, softened
- 3/4 cup brown sugar
- 21/4 cups cake flour

|Directions|

- Switch on the oven, then set it to 325 degrees F and let it preheat.
- Place butter in a bowl, add brown sugar in it, and then beat with an electric whisker until soft and fluffy.
- Then gradually stir in flour until incorporated and knead until smooth dough ball comes together.
- Place dough onto a clean and flour-dusted working space, then roll the dough into ¼-inch thick crust and then cut out diamond shape cookies with a knife or a cookie cutter.
- Take a cookie sheet, grease it with oil, place cookies in it, and bake for 10 minutes until nicely golden brown.

- When done, let cookies cool on a wire rack and then serve.

Nutrition Information –

129 Cal; 15 g Carb; 1 g Protein; 8 g Fat, 0 g Fiber; 91 mg Sodium; 38 mg Potassium; 12 mg Phosphorus;

Bagel with Egg and Salmon

|Preparation Time: 10 minutes|

|Cooking Time: 5 minutes|

|Total Time: 15 minutes|

|Serve – 1|

|Ingredients|

- 1 ounce of cooked salmon
- 1/2 of a bagel
- 1 slice of tomato
- 1/2 teaspoon fresh dill
- 4 pieces of arugula
- 2 basil leaves
- 1 tablespoon chopped scallions
- 1 tablespoon cream cheese, softened
- 1 egg

|Directions|

- Cut bagel in half and then toast one half of it in an oven or toaster.

- Meanwhile, place cream cheese in a bowl, add basil, scallion, and dill and stir until mixed.
- Then spread cream cheese mixture evenly on a toasted bagel and top with a tomato slice and arugula.
- Take a frying pan, place it over medium heat, grease it with oil and when hot, add egg and cook until scrambled to the desired level.
- Then push egg to one side of the pan, add salmon into the pan and cook for 2 minutes until warm through.
- Spoon salmon and scrambled egg on top of tomato slice and serve.

Nutrition Information –

318 Cal; 29 g Carb; 19 g Protein; 14 g Fat, 2.6 g Fiber; 378 mg Sodium; 338 mg Potassium; 270 mg Phosphorus;

Berry Smoothie Bowl

|Preparation Time: 5 minutes|

|Cooking Time: 0 minutes|

|Total Time: 5 minutes|

|Serve – 2|

|Ingredients|

- 1/4 of fresh pear, sliced

- 2 tablespoons frozen blueberries
- 1 teaspoon chia seeds
- 1 cup mixed frozen berries, unsweetened
- 3/4 cup Greek yogurt
- 1/2 cup rice milk, unsweetened
- 2 tablespoons frozen raspberries
- 1 packet of frozen acai, unsweetened

|Directions|

- Break acai into pieces, transfer it into a blender, and then add remaining ingredients, reserving pears, raspberries, and blueberries.
- Pulse the ingredients for 2 minutes until smooth and creamy, and then distribute evenly between two bowls.
- Evenly top with pears, raspberries, and blueberries and serve.

Nutrition Information –

192Cal; 28 g Carb; 11 g Protein; 4 g Fat, 7.2 g Fiber; 82 mg Sodium; 349 mg Potassium; 140 mg Phosphorus;

Apple and Onion Omelet

|Preparation Time: 10 minutes|

|Cooking Time: 22 minutes|

|Total Time: 32 minutes|

|Serve – 2|

|Ingredients|

- 1 large apple, peeled, cored, diced
- 3/4 cup sweet onion, sliced
- 1/8 teaspoon freshly cracked black pepper
- 1 tablespoon unsalted butter
- 1 tablespoon water
- 3 pasteurized eggs
- 1/4 cup almond milk
- 2 tablespoons shredded cheddar cheese, sodium-reduced

|Directions|

- Switch on the oven, then set it to 400 degrees F and let it preheat.
- Meanwhile, crack eggs in a bowl, add black pepper, water, and milk and whisk until combined, set aside until required.
- Take a medium ovenproof skillet pan, place it over medium heat, add butter and when it melts, add onion and apple and cook for 5 to 6 minutes or until softened.
- Spread onion and apple evenly in the skillet pan, pour prepared egg mixture over the vegetables, and continue cooking for 3 minutes or until edges begin to set.
- Then remove the pan from heat, top omelet with cheese, and bake for 10 to 12 minutes until the center is set.

- When done, cut omelet in half, then slide each half to a plate and serve.

Nutrition Information –

284 Cal; 22 g Carb; 13 g Protein; 16 g Fat, 3.5 g Fiber; 169 mg Sodium; 341 mg Potassium; 238 mg Phosphorus;

Asparagus and Cauliflower Tortilla

|Preparation Time: 10 minutes|

|Cooking Time: 30 minutes|

|Total Time: 40 minutes|

|Serve – 4|

|Ingredients|

- 2 cups cauliflower florets, chopped
- 11/2 cups chopped white onion
- 2 cups asparagus, chopped
- 1/2 teaspoon minced garlic
- 1/2 teaspoon freshly cracked black pepper
- 1/4 teaspoon salt
- 1/4 teaspoon ground nutmeg
- 1/4 teaspoon dried thyme, crumbled
- 2 tablespoons parsley, chopped
- 2 teaspoons olive oil

- 1 cup liquid egg substitute, low-cholesterol
- 1 tablespoon water

|Directions|

- Cut cauliflower and asparagus into bite-size pieces, then place them in a heatproof bowl, drizzle with water and microwave for 3 to 5 minutes until vegetables are tender-crisp and steamed.
- Then place a skillet pan over medium heat, add oil and when hot, add onion and cook for 7 minutes.
- Add garlic, cook for 1 minute until fragrant, switch heat to the low level, add steamed asparagus and cauliflower, season with black pepper, salt, nutmeg, thyme, and parsley, and cook for 10 to 15 minutes until the bottom has browned and the tortilla has set.
- Run a knife along the sides of pan to loosen tortilla, then transfer it to a plate by inverting it over a plate, cut it into four slices and serve.

Nutrition Information –

102 Cal; 9 g Carb; 9 g Protein; 3 g Fat, 3.88 g Fiber; 248 mg Sodium; 472 mg Potassium; 97 mg Phosphorus;

Clam Omelet

|Preparation Time: 5 minutes|

|Cooking Time: 7 minutes|

|Total Time: 12 minutes|

|Serve – 3|

|Ingredients|

- 1/4 cup clams, shelled
- 2 teaspoons cornstarch
- 2 tablespoons olive oil
- 11/2 tablespoons sweet and sour sauce
- 5 pasteurized eggs

|Directions|

- Take a large bowl, crack eggs in it, whisk with a fork until beaten, then add clam and cornstarch and stir until mixed.
- Place a skillet pan over low heat, add oil and when hot, pour in egg mixture, spread it evenly, and cook for 5 minutes until eggs are no longer runny.
- Then remove the pan from heat, cut the omelet into three portions, slide each portion onto a plate, top with sauce, and serve.

Nutrition Information –

229 Cal; 6 g Carb; 13 g Protein; 17 g Fat, 0 g Fiber; 265 mg Sodium; 132 mg Potassium; 203 mg Phosphorus;

Cheese Pancakes with Strawberries

|Preparation Time: 10 minutes|

|Cooking Time: 40 minutes|

|Total Time: 50 minutes|

|Serve – 6|

|Ingredients|

- 3 cups fresh strawberries, sliced
- 1/2 cup all-purpose white flour
- 6 tablespoons unsalted butter, melted
- 1 cup cottage cheese, sodium-reduced
- 4 pasteurized eggs, beaten

|Directions|

- Crack eggs in a bowl, whisk with a fork until beaten, add flour, butter, and cheese and stir until well combined and smooth.
- Take a frying pan, place it over medium-high heat, spray it with oil and when hot, ladle ¼ cup of prepared batter in it, shape it into 4-inches round pancake, add more batter until the pan is full and cook the pancake for 3 minutes per side until lightly browned.

- Transfer pancakes to a plate and then continue cooking more pancakes, in the same manner, about 12.
- Serve pancakes with sliced strawberries.

Nutrition Information –

253 Cal; 21 g Carb; 11 g Protein; 17 g Fat, 2 g Fiber; 172 mg Sodium; 217 mg Potassium; 159 mg Phosphorus;

Cottage Cheese and Sour Cream Pancakes

|Preparation Time: 10 minutes|

|Cooking Time: 15 minutes|

|Total Time: 25 minutes|

|Serve – 4|

|Ingredients|

- 1/2 cup all-purpose white flour
- 1/8 teaspoon salt
- 2 pasteurized eggs
- 1/2 cup cottage cheese, sodium-reduced
- 1/2 cup sour cream

|Directions|

- Prepare the batter and for this, crack eggs in a bowl, and whisk with a fork until beaten.

- Add salt, cheese, and sour cream, stir until well combined and smooth and then fold in the flour until incorporated.
- Take a frying pan, place it over medium-high heat, spray it with oil and when hot, ladle ¼ cup of prepared batter in it, shape it into 4-inches round pancake, add more batter until the pan is full and cook the pancake for 3 minutes per side until lightly browned.
- Transfer pancakes to a plate and then continue cooking more pancakes, in the same manner, about 8.
- Serve straight away.

Nutrition Information –

165 Cal; 13 g Carb; 8 g Protein; 9 g Fat; 0.4 g Fiber; 150 mg Sodium; 111 mg Potassium; 134 mg Phosphorus;

Egg and Sausage Breakfast Sandwich

|Preparation Time: 5 minutes|

|Cooking Time: 3 minutes|

|Total Time: 8 minutes|

|Serve – 1|

|Ingredients|

- 1 turkey sausage patty
- 1/4 cup liquid egg substitute, low-cholesterol
- 1 tablespoon shredded cheddar cheese, sodium-reduced
- 1 English muffin, halved, toasted

|Directions|

- Place a skillet pan over medium-low heat, spray it with oil and when hot, pour in the egg, and cook for 3 minutes until thoroughly cooked.
- Meanwhile, place the sausage patty on a heatproof plate, cover it with a paper towel and microwave for 1 minute or more until hot.
- Assemble the sandwich and for this, place sausage patty on top of the bottom half of muffin, top with cheese, then cover with the top half of muffin and serve.

Nutrition Information –

253 Cal; 26 g Carb; 17 g Protein; 9 g Fat, 2 g Fiber; 591 mg Sodium; 218 mg Potassium; 158 mg Phosphorus;

Stuffed French Toast

|Preparation Time: 5 minutes|

|Cooking Time: 12 minutes|

|Total Time: 17 minutes|

|Serve – 1|

|Ingredients|

- 2 slices of whole-wheat bread
- ½ teaspoon cinnamon
- 1-ounce softened cream cheese
- 1/4 cup liquid egg substitute, low-cholesterol
- 2 tablespoons applesauce, unsweetened

|Directions|

- Place a skillet pan over medium-high heat, grease it with oil and let it heat until hot.
- Pour in half of the egg white in a shallow dish, top with a slice of bread, let it soak and transfer bread slice into the hot pan, egg side down.
- Spread cream cheese on top of bread, add applesauce and then sprinkle with cinnamon.
- Soak remaining bread slice into the remaining egg in the same manner, then place it on top of apple sauce, egg side up, and cook for 4 to 5 minutes per side until nicely brown, flipping the toast halfway through.
- When done, transfer French toast to a plate, drizzle with maple syrup and serve.

Nutrition Information –

276 Cal; 26 g Carb; 16 g Protein; 12 g Fat, 5.4 g Fiber; 466 mg Sodium; 314 mg Potassium; 158 mg Phosphorus;

Corn Cakes with Cheese

|Preparation Time: 15 minutes|

|Cooking Time: 8 minutes|

|Total Time: 23 minutes|

|Serve – 4|

|Ingredients|

- 1/2 teaspoon anise
- 2/3 cup white corn flour
- 1 teaspoon unsalted butter
- 4 ounces Costeño cheese, sodium-reduced, grated
- 1 cup hot water

|Directions|

- Place flour in a bowl, add anise, and cheese, stir until mixed, and then slowly stir in warm water until well combined.
- Let the mixture rest for 10 minutes at room temperature, then knead for 3 minutes and shape the mixture into four 4-inches wide and ½-inch thick cakes.
- Take a skillet pan, place it over medium heat, add butter and when it melts, add corn cakes and cook for 3 minutes per side until browned.
- Serve straight away.

Nutrition Information –

285 Cal; 40 g Carb; 9 g Protein; 11 g Fat, 3.7 g Fiber; 409 mg Sodium; 198 mg Potassium; 344 mg Phosphorus;

Potato Gratin

|Preparation Time: 10 minutes|

|Cooking Time: 33 minutes|

|Total Time: 43 minutes|

|Serve – 12|

|Ingredients|

- 1 ½ teaspoon minced garlic
- 1 ¼ pound white potato, peeled, sliced
- 2 tablespoons all-purpose flour
- 1/4 teaspoon freshly cracked black pepper
- 2 tablespoons unsalted butter
- 1 cup almond milk
- 3/4 cup grated Parmesan cheese, sodium-reduced

|Directions|

- Switch on the oven, then set it to 400 degrees F and let it preheat.
- Place a small saucepan over medium heat, add butter and when it melts, add garlic and cook for 1 minute until fragrant.

- Stir in flour, cook for 1 minute, slowly whisk in milk until smooth, cook for 5 minutes and then remove the pan from heat.
- Add ½ cup cheese into the pan, stir until cheese has melted, season with black pepper and set aside until required.
- Take a twelve cups muffin tray, grease it with oil, stack potato slices in them, drizzle sauce over the top, sprinkle with remaining cheese and bake for 25 minutes.
- Let potato gratin cool for 5 minutes, then run a knife along the sides of each muffin cups to lose potatoes and transfer potato gratin to a plate.
- Serve immediately.

Nutrition Information –

98 Cal; 13 g Carb; 3 g Protein; 4 g Fat, 0.8 g Fiber; 103 mg Sodium; 228 mg Potassium; 77 mg Phosphorus;

Old Fashion Waffles

|Preparation Time: 10 minutes|

|Cooking Time: 45 minutes|

|Total Time: 55 minutes|

|Serve – 8|

|Ingredients|

- 2 cups all-purpose white flour
- 1 tablespoon coconut sugar
- 1 teaspoon salt
- 1 1/2 teaspoons nutritional yeast
- 8 tablespoons unsalted butter, cut into 8 pieces
- 1 teaspoon almond extract, unsweetened
- 2 pasteurized eggs
- 1 3/4 cups almond milk

|Directions|

- Take a small saucepan, place it over medium-low heat, pour in milk, add butter and cook for 5 minutes until it melts, set aside until cooled.
- Then place flour in a bowl, add salt, sugar, and yeasts, stir until mixed, and then whisk in milk mixture until smooth.
- Crack eggs in a bowl, whisk in vanilla, then add into the flour batter, whisk until incorporated, cover the top with plastic wrap and refrigerator for a minimum of 12 hours.
- When ready to cook, switch on the oven, then set it to 200 degrees F and let it preheat to keep waffles warm.
- Switch on the 7-inch waffle iron, then spray it with oil and let it preheat.
- Remove waffles batter from the refrigerator, stir well, then ladle ½ cup of the batter into heated waffle iron and cook for 5 minutes until firm and crispy.

- Use remaining batter for cooking seven more waffles and then serve.

Nutrition Information –

263 Cal; 25 g Carb; 7 g Protein; 15 g Fat, 0.9 g Fiber; 308 mg Sodium; 151 mg Potassium; 113 mg Phosphorus;

Spaghetti-Basil Frittata

|Preparation Time: 5 minutes|

|Cooking Time: 12 minutes|

|Total Time: 17 minutes|

|Serve – 4|

|Ingredients|

- 21/2 cups whole-wheat spaghetti, cooked
- 1/3 cup chopped green onion
- 1/4 teaspoon freshly cracked black pepper
- 2 tablespoons chopped fresh basil
- 2 teaspoons olive oil
- 4 pasteurized eggs
- 2 pasteurized egg whites
- 1/3 cup milk
- 2 ounces shredded mozzarella cheese, sodium-reduced

|Directions|

- Take a skillet pan, place it over medium heat, add oil and when hot, add spaghetti, spread it evenly, and cook for 2 minutes.
- Crack eggs in a bowl, add egg white, black pepper, and milk, whisk until blended and then pour this mixture over spaghetti.
- Sprinkle cheese on top of the frittata, top with onion and basil and cook for 8 minutes until set, covering the pan.
- When done, cut the frittata into four wedges and serve,

Nutrition Information –

271 Cal; 26 g Carb; 17 g Protein; 11 g Fat, 3.1 g Fiber; 208 mg Sodium; 212 mg Potassium; 279 mg Phosphorus;

Strawberry and Cream Cheese French Toast Casserole

|Preparation Time: 8 hours and 10 minutes|

|Cooking Time: 50 minutes|

|Total Time: 9 hours|

|Serve – 12|

|Ingredients|

- 2 cups fresh strawberries, sliced
- 1/3 cup maple syrup

- 3/4 cup coconut sugar
- 12 ounces cream cheese, cold, cut into cubes
- 2 teaspoons unsalted butter
- 9 pasteurized eggs
- 1 1/2 cups half-and-half creamer
- 12 slices of bread, Texas toast-style, cut into cubes

|Directions|

- Take a heatproof baking dish, about 9 by 13 inches in size, spray it with oil, and layer the bottom with half of the bread cubes.
- Then spread cream cheese cubes on top, layer with 1 cup sliced strawberries, and top with remaining bread cubes.
- Crack eggs in a bowl, add maple syrup and half-and-half, whisk until combined, pour this mixture over bread cubes, press the bread cubes gently to moisten them completely, then cover the bowl with plastic wrap and refrigerate for 8 hours.
- When ready to cook, switch on the oven, then set to 350 degrees F and let it preheat.
- Remove casserole from the refrigerator, uncover it and bake for 45 to 50 minutes until the top is nicely golden and inserted a knife into the center of the bread comes out clean.
- Meanwhile, prepare the sauce and for this, place remaining sliced berries in a bowl,

sprinkle with sugar, and let berries stand for 20 minutes, stirring occasionally.
- Transfer berries mixture into a blender, pulse for 2 minutes until smooth and then pour the berries mixture into a saucepan.
- Place the saucepan over medium heat, add butter, stir and cook for 5 minutes until the butter has melted, stirring occasionally, and then set aside until required.
- When casserole has cooked, remove it from the oven, let it cool for 5 minutes and then cut into twelve portions.
- Serve toast casserole with prepared strawberry sauce.

Nutrition Information –

383 Cal; 44 g Carb; 11 g Protein; 19 g Fat, 1.6 g Fiber; 358 mg Sodium; 241 mg Potassium; 179 mg Phosphorus;

Wheat and Berry Breakfast Bowl

|Preparation Time: 10 minutes|

|Cooking Time: 1 hour and 10 minutes|

|Total Time: 1 hour and 20 minutes|

|Serve – 4|

|Ingredients|

- 1 medium fresh pear, sliced
- 1/2 cup fresh cranberries
- 1/2 cups wheat berries, uncooked
- 2 tablespoons maple syrup
- 2 tablespoons crystallized ginger
- 1/2 teaspoon cinnamon
- 1 teaspoon orange zest
- 1 tablespoon unsalted butter
- 1 ½ cup water

|Directions|

- Take a saucepan, place it over medium-high heat, pour in water, add wheat berries, and bring the mixture to boil.
- Switch heat to medium-low level, and then simmer for 50 minutes until tender, covering the pan, set aside until required.
- Then place a skillet pan over medium heat, add butter and when it melts, add pear slices and cook for 5 to 8 minutes until tender.
- Add ginger and cranberries, stir and cook for 3 to 5 minutes until berries start to burst.
- Add cooked wheat berries into the pan, season with cinnamon and orange zest, drizzle with maple syrup, stir until mixed and cook for 3 minutes until thoroughly heated.
- Serve straight away.

Nutrition Information –

174 Cal; 36 g Carb; 3 g Protein; 2 g Fat, 5.1 g Fiber; 19 mg Sodium; 220 mg Potassium; 90 mg Phosphorus;

Cranberry and Roasted Garlic Risotto

|Preparation Time: 10 minutes|

|Cooking Time: 42 minutes|

|Total Time: 52 minutes|

|Serve – 4|

|Ingredients|

- 3/4 cup Arborio rice, uncooked
- 1/2 cup dried cranberries, sweetened
- 1 cup minced white onion
- 3 tablespoons roasted garlic
- 2 tablespoons unsalted butter
- 2 cups chicken broth
- 1/2 tablespoon grated Parmesan cheese, sodium-reduced

|Directions|

- Switch on the oven, then set it to 425 degrees F and let it preheat.
- Meanwhile, place a large saucepan over medium heat, add butter and when it melts,

add onion and garlic, cook for 8 minutes or until softened, add rice, stir well and continue cooking for 2 minutes.
- Add cranberries, pour in water, stir until mixed, bring the mixture to boil, then switch heat to the low level and cook for 2 minutes.
- Take a casserole dish, spray it with oil, pour in cooked onion-cranberries mixture in it, cover with aluminum foil and let it bake for 30 minutes.
- When done, unwrap the casserole, sprinkle cheese on top and serve immediately.

Nutrition Information –

267 Cal; 43 g Carb; 8 g Protein; 7 g Fat, 3 g Fiber; 100 mg Sodium; 184 mg Potassium; 66 mg Phosphorus;

Zucchini Frittata

|Preparation Time: 10 minutes|

|Cooking Time: 30 minutes|

|Total Time: 40 minutes|

|Serve – 9|

|Ingredients|

- 1 cup baking mix
- 1 medium white onion, peeled, chopped
- 3 cups grated zucchini

- 1/4 cup chopped parsley
- ½ teaspoon minced garlic
- Cracked black pepper to taste
- 1/2 teaspoon dried marjoram
- 1/2 cup canola oil
- 4 pasteurized eggs, beaten
- 1/2 cup grated parmesan cheese, sodium-reduced

|Directions|

- Switch on the oven, then set it to 350 degrees F and let it preheat.
- Meanwhile, place all the ingredients in a large bowl and then stir until mixed.
- Take an 11 by 7 inches casserole dish, spray it with oil, spoon in the prepared mixture, spread it evenly and cake for 30 minutes or until set and the top has nicely browned.
- When done, let frittata cool for 5 minutes, then cut it into nine sections and serve.

Nutrition Information –

230 Cal; 11 g Carb; 6 g Protein; 18 g Fat, 1.1 g Fiber; 260 mg Sodium; 198 mg Potassium; 107 mg Phosphorus;

Zucchini Pancakes

|Preparation Time: 10 minutes|

|Cooking Time: 10 minutes|

|Total Time: 20 minutes|

|Serve – 4|

|Ingredients|

- 1 tablespoon all-purpose white flour
- 2 cups grated zucchini
- 1/4 cup grated white onion
- 1/8 teaspoon salt
- 1 teaspoon garlic and herb seasoning, salt-free
- 1 tablespoon canola oil
- 1/4 cup liquid egg substitute, low-cholesterol

|Directions|

- Place grated zucchini and onion in a bowl, stir until combined, then wrap zucchini mixture in a kitchen towel and twist well to squeeze moisture as much as possible.
- Transfer zucchini mixture into a bowl, add remaining ingredients, except for oil, stir well until combined, and then shape the mixture into four patties.
- Take a large frying pan, place it over high heat, add oil and when hot, switch heat to medium-

low level, add patties in the pan and cook for 5 minutes per side until nicely browned.
- Serve straight away.

Nutrition Information –

55 Cal; 4 g Carb; 2 g Protein; 4 g Fat, 1 g Fiber; 89 mg Sodium; 198 mg Potassium; 27 mg Phosphorus;

Lunch

Deviled Green Beans

|Preparation Time: 10 minutes|

|Cooking Time: 1 minute|

|Total Time: 11 minutes|

|Serve – 4|

|Ingredients|

- 2 cups frozen green beans
- 1/2 teaspoon freshly cracked black pepper
- 2 teaspoons mustard
- 1 teaspoon Worcestershire sauce
- 5 teaspoons unsalted margarine, melted
- 1 tablespoon seasoned breadcrumbs

|Directions|

- Prepare the green beans, and for this, follow all the directions on its packages and set aside until required.
- Prepare the sauce and for this, place 2 teaspoons margarine in a large heatproof bowl, add black pepper, mustard and Worcestershire sauce, whisk until combined, and then heat in the microwave for 30 seconds.

- Add green beans into the sauce, toss until well mixed and then set aside until required.
- Place breadcrumbs in a small bowl, add remaining margarine in it, stir until mixed, then top the mixture over green beans and serve.

Nutrition Information –

71 Cal; 6 g Carb; 1 g Protein; 5 g Fat, 2.1 g Fiber; 92 mg Sodium; 131 mg Potassium; 23 mg Phosphorus;

Cranberry Cabbage

|Preparation Time: 5 minutes; Cooking Time: 10 minutes; Total Time: 15 minutes|

|Serve – 8|

|Ingredients|

- 1 medium head of red cabbage, shredded
- 10 ounces whole-berry cranberry sauce
- 1/4 teaspoon ground cloves
- 1 tablespoon lemon juice

|Directions|

- Take a large pan, place it over medium heat, add cloves in it, pour in lemon juice and cranberry sauce, stir until mixed and bring the sauce to simmer.

- Add cabbage into the sauce, toss until well mixed, bring the mixture to boil, then switch heat to medium-low level and continue cooking for 5 minutes or until cabbage is tender.
- Serve immediately.

Nutrition Information –

73 Cal; 18 g Carb; 1 g Protein; 0 g Fat, 1.6 g Fiber; 32 mg Sodium; 138 mg Potassium; 18 mg Phosphorus;

Buffalo Chicken Dip

|Preparation Time: 10 minutes|

|Cooking Time: 3 hours|

|Total Time: 3 hours and 10 minutes|

|Serve – 16|

|Ingredients|

- 2 cups cooked, shredded chicken
- 1/2 cup jarred roasted red peppers
- 4 teaspoons Tabasco sauce
- 1 cup sour cream
- 4 ounces softened cream cheese
- Sliced vegetables, for serving

|Directions|

- Drain the red pepper, reserving ½ cup liquid, then add the liquid and peppers into a food processor and pulse for 2 minutes until smooth.
- Place cream cheese in a bowl, add sour cream and mix well until smooth.
- Then add red pepper mixture, drizzle with 2 teaspoons of Tabasco sauce, stir until combined, add chicken and mix well.
- Stir in remaining hot pepper sauce, then spoon the mixture into a slow cooker, cover with the lid and cook for 3 hours at low heat setting.
- When done, transfer dip to a bowl and serve with sliced vegetables or serve as a lettuce wrap by wrapping dip into lettuce leaves.

Nutrition Information –

73 Cal; 2 g Carb; 5 g Protein; 5 g Fat, 0 g Fiber; 66 mg Sodium; 81 mg Potassium; 47 mg Phosphorus;

Tortilla Pizza

|Preparation Time: 10 minutes|

|Cooking Time: 15 minutes|

|Total Time: 25 minutes|

|Serve – 2|

|Ingredients|

- 2 ounces grilled chicken
- 1/4 cup sliced fresh mushrooms
- 1/4 cup chopped broccoli florets
- 1/4 cup sliced red onion
- 2 ounces cream cheese, softened
- 4 tablespoons marinara sauce
- 2 flour tortillas, each about 8-inch

|Directions|

- Switch on the oven, then set it to 400 degrees F and let it preheat.
- Then take a baking tray, line it with aluminum foil, place tortillas on it, spray with butter on both sides and bake for 10 minutes until nicely golden, flipping the tortilla halfway through
- When done, spread 1 ounce of cream cheese on top of each tortilla, then spread with 2 tablespoons of marinara sauce, top with chicken, mushroom, broccoli, and onion.
- Return tortillas into the oven, continue baking for 5 minutes or until vegetables have cooked, then cut tortillas into quarters and serve.

Nutrition Information –

326 Cal; 35 g Carb; 15 g Protein; 14 g Fat, 2.4 g Fiber; 572 mg Sodium; 397 mg Potassium; 194 mg Phosphorus;

Vegetarian Pizza

|Preparation Time: 10 minutes|

|Cooking Time: 14 minutes|

|Total Time: 24 minutes|

|Serve – 8|

|Ingredients|

- 1 pizza dough
- 1/2 cup diced red onion
- 1/2 cup chopped green bell pepper
- 1/2 cup sliced mushroom
- 1/2 cup pineapple tidbits
- 1/2 cup shredded mozzarella cheese, sodium-reduced, part-skim
- 2 tablespoons grated parmesan cheese
- 1 cup roasted red pepper tomato sauce, low-sodium

|Directions|

- Switch on the oven, then set it to 425 degrees F and let it preheat.
- Meanwhile, dough the pizza dough into two-crust, about 12-inches wide, and then spread ½ of tomato sauce on top of each crust and then scatter with onion, bell pepper, mushroom, and pineapple.

- Cover the top of the pizza with mozzarella and parmesan cheese and bake for 14 to 16 minutes until cheese has melted and pizza is cooked.
- When done, cut the pizza into slices and serve.

Nutrition Information –

289 Cal; 37 g Carb; 8 g Protein; 12 g Fat, 2.2 g Fiber; 165 mg Sodium; 210 mg Potassium; 111 mg Phosphorus;

Chiles Rellenos

|Preparation Time: 15 minutes|

|Cooking Time: 15 minutes|

|Total Time: 30 minutes|

|Serve – 3|

|Ingredients|

- 1 teaspoon minced white onion
- 1/4 cup fresh mushrooms, sliced
- 1 tablespoon minced carrot
- 2 green chili peppers
- 1 teaspoon all-purpose white flour
- 4 ounces cream cheese
- 1 egg white
- 1 cup canola oil

|Directions|

- Take a large bowl, place onion, mushrooms and carrot in it, add cream cheese stir well and let the mixture refrigerate until required.
- Take a frying pan, place it over medium heat and when hot, add peppers and cook for 3 to 5 minutes until roasted and skin bubbles, turning peppers frequently in the pan.
- Then remove the pan from heat, cool the peppers for 10 minutes, peel the skin, cut the pepper in half lengthwise and stuff the inside with prepared cream cheese mixture.
- Place egg white in a shallow dish, whisk until flour until combined and stiff batter comes together, and then coat stuffed peppers in it.
- Place a saucepan over medium-high heat, pour in the oil, and when hot, add stuffed peppers in it and cook for 5 to 8 minutes until golden brown, turning once.
- Transfer fried peppers to a plate lined with paper towels and serve.

Nutrition Information –

304 Cal; 6 g Carb; 7 g Protein; 28 g Fat, 1.3 g Fiber; 259 mg Sodium; 244 mg Potassium; 58 mg Phosphorus;

Pasta Primavera

|Preparation Time: 10 minutes|

|Cooking Time: 20 minutes|

|Total Time: 30 minutes|

|Serve – 6|

|Ingredients|

- 12 ounces penne pasta, cooked
- 2 tablespoons all-purpose white flour
- 12 ounces of frozen mixed vegetables, cooked
- 1/4 teaspoon garlic powder
- 1/4 cup half-and-half creamer
- 14 ounces chicken broth
- 1/4 cup grated Parmesan cheese

|Directions|

- Place a medium stockpot over low heat, pour in the broth, then whisk in flour until combined, add garlic powder and creamer and stir until mixed.
- Simmer the soup for 10 minutes until slightly thickened, then add pasta and vegetables, stir well and cook for 5 to 10 minutes until thoroughly heated.
- Ladle pasta and vegetables into dishes, top with cheese, and serve.

Nutrition Information –

273 Cal; 48 g Carb; 13 g Protein; 3 g Fat, 4.5 g Fiber; 115 mg Sodium; 251 mg Potassium; 154 mg Phosphorus;

Tempeh Pita Sandwiches

|Preparation Time: 10 minutes|

|Cooking Time: 20 minutes|

|Total Time: 30 minutes|

|Serve – 4|

|Ingredients|

- 8 ounces tempeh
- 1/2 cup sliced mushrooms
- 1 red bell pepper, cored, sliced
- 1 small white onion, peeled, sliced
- 2 tablespoons balsamic vinegar
- 2 tablespoons sesame oil
- 4 teaspoons mayonnaise
- 2 pieces of pita bread, about 6-inch

|Directions|

- Take a large skillet pan, place it over medium heat, add 1 tablespoon oil and let it heat until hot.

- Cut tempeh into twelve slices, add to the skillet pan and cook for 3 to 4 minutes per side until browned.
- Drizzle vinegar over tempeh, cook for 1 minute, then flip and cook for another minute.
- Transfer tempeh slices to a plate, add remaining oil into the pan, switch heat to medium level, then add pepper, onion, and mushroom and cook for 5 to 8 minutes until tender.
- Assemble sandwiches and for this, cut the pita bread in half, open its pocket, then spread 1 teaspoon mayonnaise into each pitta pocket and stiff with three tempeh slices and ¼ of the cooked vegetable mixture.
- Serve straight away.

Nutrition Information –

313 Cal; 25 g Carb; 15 g Protein; 17 g Fat, 5.5 g Fiber; 187 mg Sodium; 437 mg Potassium; 208 mg Phosphorus;

Triple Berry Salad

|Preparation Time: 10 minutes|

|Cooking Time: 20 minutes|

|Total Time: 30 minutes|

|Serve – 4|

|Ingredients|

- 2 cups fresh strawberries, rinsed, sliced
- 1 cup fresh blackberries, rinsed
- 1 cup fresh blueberries, rinsed
- 1/8 teaspoon cinnamon
- 2 cups cottage cheese, sodium-reduced
- 1/4 cup lemon juice

|Directions|

- Take a salad bowl, place sliced strawberries in it, add remaining berries, drizzle with lemon juice, and toss until well mixed.
- Distribute cottage cheese between four plates, top with berries, sprinkle with cinnamon, and serve.

Nutrition Information –

140 Cal; 15 g Carb; 15 g Protein; 2 g Fat, 4.3 g Fiber; 382 mg Sodium; 350 mg Potassium; 181 mg Phosphorus;

Veggie Strata

|Preparation Time: 1 hour and 15 minutes|

|Cooking Time: 1 hour and 20 minutes|

|Total Time: 2 hours and 35 minutes|

|Serve – 9|

|Ingredients|

- 7 slices of sourdough bread, each about ½-inch thick
- 1 cup diced white onion
- 15 spinach leaves, fresh
- 1 cup diced mushrooms
- 1 cup diced red bell peppers
- 1/2 teaspoon freshly cracked black pepper
- 1/4 cup tarragon vinegar
- 1 teaspoon Tabasco sauce
- 1 teaspoon Worcestershire sauce
- 1 tablespoon unsalted margarine
- 1-ounce shredded sharp cheddar cheese, sodium-reduced
- 7 pasteurized eggs
- 13/4 cups half-and-half creamer

|Directions|

- Switch on the oven, then set it to 225 degrees F and let it preheat.
- Then cut bread slices into cubes, spread them on a baking sheet, and bake for 30 minutes until crispy and dry, turning halfway through.
- Place a small skillet pan over medium heat, add margarine and when it melts, add red pepper, mushroom, and onion and cook for 5 minutes until tender.
- Take a 9-inch baking dish, grease it oil, spread half of the bread cubes in a single in its bottom,

and top with half of the cooked vegetable mixture.
- Layer vegetables with spinach leaves, scatter with remaining bread cubes, and then top with remaining vegetable mixture.
- Crack eggs in a bowl, add black pepper, vinegar, hot sauce, Worcestershire sauce, and creamer, whisk until well combined, and then evenly pour this mixture over bread cubes.
- Cover the casserole dish with plastic wrap and then place it into the refrigerator for a minimum of 1 hour.
- Then let the casserole stand for 20 minutes and in the meantime, set the oven to 325 degrees F and let it preheat.
- Unwrap the casserole, bake it for 50 minutes until top is nicely golden brown, then top with cheese and continue cooking for 10 minutes until cheese has melted and a knife inserted into the center of the dish comes out clean.
- When done, cut strata into nine portions and serve immediately.

Nutrition Information –

212 Cal; 15 g Carb; 11 g Protein; 12 g Fat, 2 g Fiber; 218 mg Sodium; 347 mg Potassium; 207 mg Phosphorus;

Buffalo Wings

|Preparation Time: 10 minutes|

|Cooking Time: 35 minutes|

|Total Time: 45 minutes|

|Serve – 12|

|Ingredients|

- 24 chicken wing drumettes
- 1/2 teaspoon garlic powder
- 1/2 teaspoon dried Italian seasoning blend
- 1/4 cup roasted red pepper sauce
- 1/3 cup Tabasco sauce
- 1/4 cup tomato sauce
- 1 tablespoon olive oil
- 8 tablespoons unsalted butter

|Directions|

- Switch on the oven, then set it to 400 degrees F and let it preheat.
- Meanwhile, place a saucepan over medium heat, add butter and when it melts, add garlic powder, Italian seasoning, red pepper sauce, Tabasco sauce and tomato sauce, and oil, and stir until combined.
- Take a baking dish, place chicken wings in it, pour prepared sauce over them, and bake for 35 minutes until done.

- Serve straight away.

Nutrition Information –

131 Cal; 0 g Carb; 8 g Protein; 11 g Fat, 0 g Fiber; 64 mg Sodium; 105 mg Potassium; 61 mg Phosphorus;

Mashed Cauliflower Potatoes

|Preparation Time: 10 minutes|

|Cooking Time: 18 minutes|

|Total Time: 28 minutes|

|Serve – 4|

|Ingredients|

- 8 ounces cauliflower florets
- 1 medium red potato, peeled
- 1/4 cup chopped white onion
- 1/4 teaspoon garlic powder
- 1 teaspoon dried parsley
- Cracked black pepper, to taste
- 2 tablespoons unsalted margarine
- Water as needed

|Directions|

- Take a large pot, add all the ingredients in it, except for water, black pepper, and margarine, and then pour in water enough to cover the vegetables.

- Place pot over high heat, bring to boil, then switch heat to medium level and simmer vegetables for 12 minutes until tender.
- Drain the vegetables, then return them into the pot, mash well with a potato masher, add margarine and stir well until smooth.
- Stir in black pepper and serve straight away.

Nutrition Information –

83 Cal; 7 g Carb; 2 g Protein; 4 g Fat, 6 g Fiber; 67 mg Sodium; 282 mg Potassium; 52 mg Phosphorus;

Potato Salad

|Preparation Time: 10 minutes|

|Cooking Time: 10 minutes|

|Total Time: 20 minutes|

|Serve – 8|

|Ingredients|

- 1 small white onion, peeled, chopped
- ½ of medium red bell pepper, chopped
- 3 medium potatoes, peeled
- 1 stalk of celery, chopped
- 1/2 teaspoon cracked black pepper
- 3 pasteurized eggs, hard-boiled
- 3 tablespoons apple cider vinegar
- 1 teaspoon Dijon mustard

- 3/4 cup mayonnaise with olive oil

|Directions|

- Cut peeled potatoes into cubes, place them in a pot, cover with water, then place the pot over high heat and bring to boil.
- Then drain potatoes, pour in freshwater, and continue boiling the potatoes until fork-tender.
- Meanwhile, prepare the vegetables and chop the eggs and set aside until required.
- When potatoes have cooked, drain them, then transfer them in a bowl, add onion, bell pepper, celery, and egg. Don't stir.
- Prepare salad dressing and for this, place vinegar, mustard, and mayonnaise in a bowl and then whisk until combined.
- Drizzle the prepared salad dressing over the salad, gently toss until mixed, then cover the bowl and chill for 30 minutes in the refrigerator.
- Serve straight away.

Nutrition Information –

172 Cal; 12 g Carb; 4 g Protein; 12 g Fat, 0.9 g Fiber; 222 mg Sodium; 213 mg Potassium; 81 mg Phosphorus;

Flavorful Grilled Salmon

|Preparation Time: 10 minutes|

|Cooking Time: 20 minutes|

|Total Time: 30 minutes|

|Serve – 6|

|Ingredients|

- 24 ounces salmon fillets, about six
- 6 slices of lemon
- 1 tablespoon capers
- 1 tablespoon fresh rosemary
- ½ teaspoon garlic and herb seasoning blend, salt-free
- ¾ cup white wine
- 6 tablespoons lemon juice
- 3 tablespoons olive oil

|Directions|

- Prepare salmon and for this, brush oil on both sides of salmon fillets and then sprinkle with the seasoning blend until well coated.
- Take six large pieces of aluminum foil, and working on one salmon at a time, place a salmon fillet on a piece of foil, top with a lemon slice, drizzle 1 tablespoon lemon juice and 2 tablespoons wine, top with ½ teaspoon capers and wrap the fillet tightly into the packets.

- Take a grill pan, place it over medium-high heat and when hot, add salmon packets on it and cook until done, 10 minutes cooking per pinch of a thick piece of salmon.
- Serve straight away.

Nutrition Information –

224 Cal; 2 g Carb; 25 g Protein; 13 g Fat, 0.2 g Fiber; 96 mg Sodium; 524 mg Potassium; 302 mg Phosphorus;

Salmon and Summer Squash

|Preparation Time: 10 minutes|

|Cooking Time: 15 minutes|

|Total Time: 25 minutes|

|Serve – 4|

|Ingredients|

- 1 pound salmon fillets
- 2 medium crookneck squash
- 1 tablespoon chopped shallot
- 1/4 teaspoon salt
- 1 teaspoon freshly cracked black pepper
- 2 tablespoons chopped dill weed
- 2 tablespoons red wine vinegar
- 3 tablespoons olive oil

|Directions|

- Prepare squash and for this, cut into ¼ by 2 ½ inch thick sticks and set aside until required.
- Prepare the salad dressing and for this, place shallots in a dressing bottle, add dill, ¼ teaspoon black pepper, vinegar, and 2 tablespoon olive oil, shake well and set aside until required.
- Prepare salmon and for this, brush it with oil, rub it well, and then season with ½ teaspoon black pepper.
- Place a skillet pan over medium heat, spray with oil, place the salmon fillet in it, skin-side down, and cook for 8 to 10 minutes until opaque and thoroughly cooked.
- Transfer salmon to a plate, then switch heat to medium-high level, add remaining oil and when hot, add squash pieces, season with salt and remaining black pepper and cook for 4 minutes until tender-crisp.
- Remove skin from each salmon fillet, then cut each fillet into four portions and distribute salmon pieces and squash between four serving dishes.
- Drizzle with prepared salad dressing and then serve.

Nutrition Information –

260 Cal; 2 g Carb; 25 g Protein; 17 g Fat, 0.9 g Fiber; 188 mg Sodium; 670 mg Potassium; 324 mg Phosphorus;

Autumn Wild Rice

|Preparation Time: 15 minutes|

|Cooking Time: 30 minutes|

|Total Time: 45 minutes|

|Serve – 8|

|Ingredients|

- 1/4 cup chopped green bell pepper
- 3/4 cup shredded carrots
- 1/4 cup chopped celery
- 2 cups chopped apples
- 1/4 teaspoon freshly cracked black pepper
- 1/4 teaspoon dried whole sage
- 2 tablespoons raisins
- 1 fresh sage sprig
- 1/4 cup fresh lemon juice
- 11/2 cups chicken broth
- 3/4 cup converted rice, uncooked
- 1/2 cup wild rice, cooked
- ¼ cup hot water

|Directions|

- Place raisins in a small bowl, pour in hot water, let raisin stand for 5 minutes, then drain well and set aside until required.
- Place a large skillet pan over medium-high heat, grease it with oil and when hot, add bell pepper, carrots, celery, and apple and cook for 3 minutes until tender-crisp, set aside until required.
- Place a large saucepan over medium-high heat, pour in chicken broth, stir in black pepper and sage and bring it to boil.
- Add converted rice, stir well and simmer for 20 minutes until rice has cooked and has absorbed all the liquid, covering the pan.
- Then remove from heat, add wild rice, apple mixture, raisin, and lemon juice, stir well until combined, and let stand for 5 minutes, covering the pan.
- Distribute rice between eight dishes, garnish with sage sprigs and serve.

Nutrition Information –

112 Cal; 24 g Carb; 4 g Protein; 0 g Fat, 1.6 g Fiber; 148 mg Sodium; 155 mg Potassium; 39 mg Phosphorus;

Gratin Pasta with Chicken and Watercress

|Preparation Time: 10 minutes|

|Cooking Time: 55 minutes|

|Total Time: 1 hour and 5 minutes|

|Serve – 4|

|Ingredients|

- 1 cup shredded, cooked chicken
- 1 small white onion, peeled, chopped
- 1 cup chopped watercress, fresh
- 1 teaspoon minced garlic
- 1/4 teaspoon freshly cracked black pepper
- 1 tablespoon olive oil
- 1 2/3 cup béchamel sauce
- 1/2 cup grated Parmesan cheese, sodium-reduced
- 2 cups pasta shells, cooked

|Directions|

- Take a skillet pan, place it over medium heat, then add oil and when hot, add onion and garlic and cook for 5 minutes or until sauté.
- Then add watercress and chicken, stir well and cook for 5 minutes until watercress is wilted.

- Transfer chicken mixture in a bowl, add pasta half of the béchamel sauce, mix well and then spoon into a greased baking dish.
- Cover pasta with remaining béchamel sauce, sprinkle with cheese and bake for 30 to 40 minutes until done and the top is nicely golden brown.
- Serve straight away.

Nutrition Information –

345 Cal; 38 g Carb; 19 g Protein; 13 g Fat; 2.1 g Fiber; 437 mg Sodium; 337 mg Potassium; 248 mg Phosphorus;

Cranberry Rice Pilaf

|Preparation Time: 50 minutes|

|Cooking Time: 12 minutes|

|Total Time: 1 hour and 2 minutes|

|Serve – 6|

|Ingredients|

- 2 tablespoons dried cranberries, sweetened
- 1/2 teaspoon black cumin
- 1 bay leaf
- 1 cinnamon stick
- 2 tablespoons unsalted butter
- 2 cups of water

- 1 cup long-grain white rice, uncooked

|Directions|

- Place rice in a pot, then add remaining ingredients and let it soak for 45 minutes at room temperature.
- Then transfer the rice mixture into a microwave rice cooker and cook for 12 minutes at full power or bring the mixture to boil and then simmer for 20 minutes.
- When done, let pilaf stand for 5 minutes and then serve.

Nutrition Information –

125 Cal; 21 g Carb; 2 g Protein; 4 g Fat, 0.7 g Fiber; 34 mg Sodium; 71 mg Potassium; 74 mg Phosphorus;

Lemon Rice with Vegetables

|Preparation Time: 10 minutes|

|Cooking Time: 35 minutes|

|Total Time: 45 minutes|

|Serve – 5|

|Ingredients|

- 1/2 cup sliced celery
- 1/4 cup chopped white onion
- 11/2 cups fresh mushrooms

- 1/8 teaspoon freshly cracked black pepper
- 1/8 teaspoon dried thyme
- 1/8 teaspoon garlic and herb seasoning, salt-free
- 1 teaspoon grated lemon zest
- 3 tablespoons unsalted margarine
- 2 tablespoons lemon juice
- 1 1/4 cups water
- 2/3 cup long-grain white rice, uncooked

|Directions|

- Take a large skillet pan, place it over medium heat, add 1 ½ tablespoon margarine and when it melts, add onion and celery and cook for 5 minutes or until sauté.
- Add black pepper, herb seasoning, thyme, lemon zest, lemon juice, and water, stir well and bring the mixture to boil.
- Then switch heat to medium-low level, add rice and simmer for 20 minutes until tender, covering the pan.
- Meanwhile, place skillet pan over medium heat, add remaining margarine and when it melts, add mushrooms and cook for 5 minutes until tender.
- Distribute rice between dishes, top with mushroom, and serve.

Nutrition Information –

183 Cal; 27 g Carb; 3 g Protein; 7 g Fat, 0.7 g Fiber; 13 mg Sodium; 143 mg Potassium; 37 mg Phosphorus;

Singapore Rice Noodles

|Preparation Time: 10 minutes|

|Cooking Time: 18 minutes|

|Total Time: 28 minutes|

|Serve – 6|

|Ingredients|

- 2 medium carrots, peeled, sliced into matchsticks
- 1 cup sliced snow peas
- 4 scallions, sliced
- 1 bunch of cilantro, chopped
- 8 ounces rice noodles, cooked
- 1/2 teaspoon garlic powder
- 1 tablespoon curry powder
- 1 tablespoon soy sauce
- 14 ounces chicken broth
- 1 tablespoon canola oil
- 2 pasteurized eggs, beaten

|Directions|

- Prepare the broth mixture and for this, place garlic powder and curry powder in a bowl, add

oil, soy sauce, and chicken broth and whisk until combined.
- Place a frying pan over high heat, pour in broth mixture, and then bring it to boil, covering the pan.
- Then switch heat to medium level, add carrots and snow peas and cook for 3 to 4 minutes until carrots have softened, and peas turn bright green.
- Remove pan from heat, add noodles and half of the cilantro, mix well, cover the pan, and set aside until required.
- Place another frying pan over medium heat, grease it with oil and when hot, pour in eggs and cook for 5 minutes until scrambled, stirring continuously.
- Chop eggs with a fork, add to noodles mixture, mix well and then distribute between six dishes.
- Garnish prepared rice noodles with remaining cilantro and scallion and then serve.

Nutrition Information –

222 Cal; 30 g Carb; 12 g Protein; 6 g Fat, 4.3 g Fiber; 216 mg Sodium; 350 mg Potassium; 194 mg Phosphorus;

Shrimp Fried Rice

|Preparation Time: 10 minutes|

|Cooking Time: 18 minutes|

|Total Time: 28 minutes|

|Serve – 4|

|Ingredients|

- 4 cups long-grain white rice, cooked, cooled
- 1/2 cup small shrimp, pre-cooked
- 3 tablespoons chopped scallions
- 1 cup frozen peas and carrots
- 3/4 cup diced white onion
- ¼ teaspoon minced garlic
- 1 tablespoon grated ginger root
- 1/4 teaspoon salt
- 3/4 teaspoon freshly cracked black pepper
- 5 tablespoons peanut oil
- 4 pasteurized eggs, beaten

|Directions|

- Place a large skillet pan over medium-high heat, add 1 tablespoon oil and when hot, add onion, season with ½ teaspoon black pepper, and cook for 2 minutes until tender.
- Add scallions, ginger, and garlic, stir well, cook for 1 minute, then add shrimps and cook for 2 minutes until hot.

- Add carrot and peas, stir, continue cooking for 2 minutes until heated, and then transfer into a large bowl, covering with the lid.
- Return skillet over medium-high heat, add 2 tablespoons oil and when hot, pour in eggs, cook for 3 minutes until scrambled and then transfer eggs to the bowl containing shrimps and vegetables.
- Return skillet pan over medium heat, add 1 tablespoon oil and when hot, add rice, stir well until coat and cook for 4 minutes until hot.
- Season rice with salt and black pepper, continue cooking for 2 minutes, add vegetables, eggs, and shrimps, stir well and cook for 2 minutes until hot.
- Serve straight away.

Nutrition Information –

421 Cal; 53 g Carb; 16 g Protein; 16 g Fat, 2.5 g Fiber; 271 mg Sodium; 285 mg Potassium; 218 mg Phosphorus;

Grilled Salmon Sandwiches

|Preparation Time: 15 minutes|

|Cooking Time: 20 minutes|

|Total Time: 35 minutes|

|Serve – 4|

|Ingredients|

- 4 slices of sourdough bread
- 4 salmon fillets, each about 4 ounces
- 1 cup arugula
- 1/2 cup diced roasted red peppers
- 1/2 teaspoon lemon-pepper seasoning
- 1 tablespoon olive oil
- 1 tablespoon lime juice
- 1/4 cup chipotle mayonnaise

|Directions|

- Set the grill and then let it preheat at a medium-high setting.
- Brush salmon with 1 tablespoon oil, rub it well, add to grill and cook for 10 to 15 minutes until fork-tender, covering the grill.
- Meanwhile, prepare the dressing and for this, place lemon pepper seasoning in a small bowl, add lemon juice and remaining oil and whisk until combined.
- When salmon has grilled, transfer it to a plate, cover salmon with foil, let it rest for 10 minutes, and then remove the skin.
- While salmon is resting, brush olive oil mixture on both sides of bread slices, then place them on the grilling rack and cook for 2 minutes per side until toasted.

- Assemble sandwich and for this, spread mayonnaise on top of bread, then top with salmon, arugula, and red pepper and serve.

Nutrition Information –

382 Cal; 20 g Carb; 26 g Protein; 22 g Fat, 1 g Fiber; 384 mg Sodium; 640 mg Potassium; 268 mg Phosphorus;

Shrimp and Broccoli Fettuccine

|Preparation Time: 10 minutes|

|Cooking Time: 22 minutes|

|Total Time: 32 minutes|

|Serve – 4|

|Ingredients|

- ¾ pound frozen medium shrimp, peeled, deveined
- 13/4 cup broccoli florets
- 1/4 cup chopped red bell pepper
- ½ teaspoon minced garlic
- 1/2 teaspoon garlic powder
- 3/4 teaspoon ground peppercorns
- 1/4 cup lemon juice
- 1 tablespoon olive oil
- 10 ounces softened cream cheese

- 1/4 cup half-and-half creamer
- 4 ounces fettuccine, uncooked

|Directions|

- Place a medium saucepan, half-full with water, over medium heat, bring it to boil, then add fettuccine and cook for 7 to 10 minutes until tender.
- Add broccoli florets in the last three minutes of cooking, cook until tender-crisp, then drain well and set aside until required, keep warm.
- Take a large skillet pan, place it over medium heat, add oil and when hot, add shrimps and minced garlic and cook for 3 minutes until thoroughly heated.
- Then add garlic powder, peppercorns, cream cheese and creamer, drizzle with lemon juice, stir well and cook for 2 minutes.
- Add pasta, toss until well mixed, then remove the pan from heat, sprinkle bell pepper on top, and serve.

Nutrition Information –

468 Cal; 28 g Carb; 27 g Protein; 28 g Fat, 2.6 g Fiber; 374 mg Sodium; 469 mg Potassium; 335 mg Phosphorus;

Fish Fry with Seasoned Rice

|Preparation Time: 10 minutes|

|Cooking Time: 28 minutes|

|Total Time: 38 minutes|

|Serve – 4|

|Ingredients|

- 1 pound frozen cod fillets, thawed
- 1 cup all-purpose white flour
- 1 cup long-grain white rice, uncooked
- 1 large white onion, peeled, diced
- 1/2 teaspoon salt
- 1 teaspoon herb seasoning blend, salt-free
- 11/2 teaspoons ground cumin
- 11/2 teaspoons freshly cracked black pepper
- 1 cup olive oil
- 2 cups of water

|Directions|

- Place pot over medium heat, add 2 teaspoon oil, and when hot, add onion and cook for 5 minutes or until sauté and browned.
- Then switch heat to medium-low level, add rice, season with ½ teaspoon each of cumin and black pepper, pour in water, stir well and cook for 20 minutes until cooked, set aside until required.

- Meanwhile, place flour in a bowl, add herb seasoning and remaining black pepper and cumin, stir until mixed and set aside until required.
- Prepare cod fillets, and for this, pat dry fillets and then dredge into the flour mixture.
- Take a skillet pan, place it over medium heat, add remaining oil and when hot, add coated fillets in it and cook for 5 minutes per side until cooked.
- Serve cod fillets with seasoned rice.

Nutrition Information –

405 Cal; 55 g Carb; 26 g Protein; 9 g Fat; 1.9 g Fiber; 360 mg Sodium; 618 mg Potassium; 316 mg Phosphorus;

Korean-Style Fried Fish

|Preparation Time: 10 minutes|

|Cooking Time: 15 minutes|

|Total Time: 25 minutes|

|Serve – 4|

|Ingredients|

- 1 pound white fish fillets
- 3 tablespoons all-purpose white flour
- 1/2 teaspoon freshly cracked black pepper

- 1 tablespoon rice vinegar, unseasoned
- 1 teaspoon soy sauce, low-sodium
- 3 tablespoons sesame oil
- 2 pasteurized eggs, beaten

|Directions|

- Rinse fish fillets, pat dry with paper towels, then cut it into 1 1/2-inch piece and set aside until required.
- Place flour in a plastic bag, add black pepper and fish pieces, seal the bag and shake well until well coated.
- Crack eggs in a bowl, then dip the fish pieces in it and set aside until required.
- Take a skillet pan, place it over medium heat, add oil and when hot, add fish pieces in a single layer and cook for 3 minutes per side until golden brown.
- Meanwhile, prepare the dressing and for this, place soy sauce and vinegar in a bowl and stir until combined.
- When done, distribute fish pieces between four dishes, drizzle with prepared dressing and serve.

Nutrition Information –

273 Cal; 4 g Carb; 26 g Protein; 17 g Fat, 0.1 g Fiber; 134 mg Sodium; 400 mg Potassium; 359 mg Phosphorus;

Pumpkin Chili

|Preparation Time: 10 minutes|

|Cooking Time: 1 hour and 18 minutes|

|Total Time: 1 hour and 28 minutes|

|Serve – 10|

|Ingredients|

- 1 cup cooked red kidney beans
- 2 pounds ground turkey, uncooked
- 1/2 cup chopped celery
- 1/2 cup sliced carrots
- 1/2 cup chopped green chilis
- 1/2 cup chopped white onion
- 1 ½ teaspoon minced garlic
- 1 tablespoon red chili powder
- 2 teaspoons cumin
- 1 teaspoon dried oregano
- 2 tablespoons olive oil
- 2 bay leaves
- 15 ounces pumpkin puree
- 3 cups chicken broth, low-sodium

|Directions|

- Take a large pot, place it over medium heat, add 1 tablespoon oil and when hot, add carrot,

celery, and onion and cook for 5 minutes until tender.
- Transfer vegetables to a plate, add remaining oil and into the pot, add turkey and cook for 8 minutes until meat is no longer pink.
- Return vegetables into the pot, add remaining ingredients, stir well until mixed, then switch heat to medium-low level and simmer the chili for 1 hour until thoroughly cooked.
- When done, remove bay leaves from chili, ladle into bowls and then serve.

Nutrition Information –

168 Cal; 7 g Carb; 24 g Protein; 5 g Fat, 3.5 g Fiber; 200 mg Sodium; 476 mg Potassium; 215 mg Phosphorus;

Chicken Noodle Soup

|Preparation Time: 10 minutes|

|Cooking Time: 25 minutes|

|Total Time: 35 minutes|

|Serve – 4|

|Ingredients|

- 1 cup chicken, cooked, shredded
- 1/4 cup diced carrot
- 1/4 teaspoon salt

- 1/4 teaspoon poultry seasoning
- 1/4 teaspoon freshly cracked black pepper
- 11/2 cups chicken broth, low-sodium
- 2 ounces egg noodles, uncooked
- 1 cup of water

|Directions|

- Pour chicken broth in a slow cooker, add water, then shut with lid and cook on high-heat setting.
- Meanwhile, prepare chicken and for this, season it with salt, black pepper, and poultry seasoning and set aside until required.
- Add chicken into the slow cooker, then add carrots and noodles, stir until mixed, and cook for 25 minutes until cooked.
- Serve straight away.

Nutrition Information –

141 Cal; 11 g Carb; 15 g Protein; 4 g Fat; 0.7 g Fiber; 191 mg Sodium; 135 mg Potassium; 104 mg Phosphorus;

Crab Cakes

|Preparation Time: 10 minutes|

|Cooking Time: 10 minutes|

|Total Time: 20 minutes|

|Serve – 6|

|Ingredients|

- 1 pound crab meat
- 1/3 cup chopped green bell pepper
- 1/4 cup chopped white onion
- 1 tablespoon garlic powder
- 1/8 teaspoon cayenne pepper
- 1 tablespoon fresh parsley
- 1 tablespoon dry mustard
- 1 teaspoon freshly cracked black pepper
- 2 tablespoons lemon juice
- 3 tablespoons olive oil
- 1 egg
- 1/4 cup mayonnaise, reduced-fat
- 6 crushed crackers, low-salt

|Directions|

- Take a large bowl, place all the ingredients in it, except for oil, stir well until mixed and then shape the mixture into six patties.
- Take a skillet pan, grease it with oil and when hot, add patties and cook for 4 minutes per side until browned.
- Serve straight away.

Nutrition Information –

188 Cal; 5 g Carb; 13 g Protein; 13 g Fat, 0.5 g Fiber; 342 mg Sodium; 317 mg Potassium; 185 mg Phosphorus;

Eggplant Seafood Casserole

|Preparation Time: 10 minutes|

|Cooking Time: 40 minutes|

|Total Time: 50 minutes|

|Serve – 8|

|Ingredients|

- 1/3 cup long-grain white rice, uncooked
- 1/2 pound boiled shrimp
- 1 pound crab meat
- 2 medium eggplant
- 1 medium white onion, peeled, chopped
- 1 medium green bell pepper, chopped
- 1/2 cup chopped celery
- 1 teaspoon minced garlic
- 1/8 teaspoon cayenne pepper
- 1/4 teaspoon Creole seasoning
- 1 tablespoon Worcestershire sauce
- 1/2 teaspoon Tabasco sauce
- 2 tablespoons unsalted butter, melted
- 1/4 cup olive oil
- 1/4 cup lemon juice

- 1/4 cup grated Parmesan cheese, sodium-reduced
- 1/2 cup breadcrumbs
- 3 pasteurized eggs

|Directions|

- Switch on the oven, then set it to 350 degrees F and let it preheat.
- Meanwhile, cut the eggplant into 1-inch pieces, place it in a medium saucepan, pour in enough water to cover eggplant and boil at medium-high heat for 5 minutes until tender.
- Then drain well, transfer eggplant into a bowl and set aside until required.
- Place a frying pan over medium heat, add oil and when hot, add celery, onion, bell pepper, and garlic and cook for 4 minutes until golden brown.
- Transfer vegetable mixture into the eggplant, add remaining ingredients except for breadcrumbs and butter, and stir until mixed.
- Take a casserole dish, grease it with oil, spoon in eggplant mixture, and spread evenly.
- Stir together breadcrumbs and butter until combined, then spread it on top of casserole and bake for 30 minutes until cooked through and the top is nicely browned.
- Serve straight away.

Nutrition Information –

216 Cal; 14 g Carb; 13 g Protein; 12 g Fat, 2.3 g Fiber; 229 mg Sodium; 359 mg Potassium; 148 mg Phosphorus;

Seafood Corn Chowder

|Preparation Time: 10 minutes|

|Cooking Time: 15 minutes|

|Total Time: 25 minutes|

|Serve – 10|

|Ingredients|

- 10 ounces crab chunks
- 2 cups frozen corn kernels
- 1/2 cup chopped green bell pepper
- 1/2 cup chopped red bell pepper
- 1 cup chopped white onion
- 1/3 cup chopped celery
- 1 tablespoon all-purpose white flour
- 1/2 teaspoon paprika
- 1/2 teaspoon freshly cracked black pepper
- 1 tablespoon unsalted butter
- 2 cups half-and-half creamer
- 6 ounces evaporated milk, unsweetened
- 14 ounces chicken broth, low-sodium

|Directions|

- Place a saucepan over medium heat, add butter and when it melts, add bell peppers, celery, and onion and then cook for 5 minutes until soft.
- Stir in flour, cook for 2 minutes, then stir in chicken broth until blended and bring the mixture to boil.
- Add corn and crab meat, season with black pepper and paprika, pour in milk and creamer, stir well and cook for 5 minutes until hot.
- Serve immediately.

Nutrition Information –

173 Cal; 22 g Carb; 8 g Protein; 7 g Fat, 1.5 g Fiber; 160 mg Sodium; 285 mg Potassium; 181 mg Phosphorus;

Dinner

Chicken Chili

|Preparation Time: 10 minutes|

|Cooking Time: 1 hour and 10 minutes|

|Total Time: 1 hour and 20 minutes|

|Serve – 8|

|Ingredients|

- 1 1/2 pounds boneless chicken, cooked, diced
- 1 cup cooked kidney beans
- 1 cup chopped white onion
- 1 cup diced tomatoes, low-sodium
- 1 cup chopped carrots
- 2 teaspoons minced garlic
- 1 cup chopped celery
- 1 cup chopped green bell pepper
- 3 tablespoons red chili powder
- 1 teaspoon dried oregano
- 1 tablespoon canola oil
- 3/4 cup tomato salsa, low-sodium
- 1/2 cup grated cheddar cheese
- 1/2 cup sour cream
- 14 ounces chicken broth, low-sodium
- 4 cups long-grain white rice, cooked

|Directions|

- Take a large pot, place it over medium heat, add oil and when hot, add onion, carrot, green pepper, celery, and garlic and cook for 8 minutes until soft.
- Pour in broth, bring it to boil, then add chicken, tomatoes, beans and salsa, season with oregano and chili powder, stir well and simmer the chili for 1 hour.
- When done, distribute rice between eight dishes, top with 1 cup chili, garnish with 1 tablespoon cheddar cheese and sour cream and then serve.

Nutrition Information –

355 Cal; 38 g Carb; 24 g Protein; 12 g Fat, 4.7 g Fiber; 348 mg Sodium; 653 mg Potassium; 270 mg Phosphorus;

Chicken Wild Rice Soup

|Preparation Time: 10 minutes|

|Cooking Time: 18 minutes|

|Total Time: 28 minutes|

|Serve – 4|

|Ingredients|

- 1/4 cup all-purpose white flour
- 8 ounces chicken breast, cooked, chopped
- 1 cup grated carrots
- 1 tablespoon minced onion
- 2/3 cup wild rice and long-grain rice blend, uncooked
- 1 tablespoon fresh parsley
- 2 tablespoons unsalted butter
- 5 cups chicken broth, low-sodium
- ½ cup of water
- 1 tablespoon slivered almonds

|Directions|

- Switch on the rice cooker, add rice blend in it, pour in 2 cups chicken broth and water, stir well, and cook until done.
- Place a saucepan over medium heat, add butter and when it melts, add onion and cook for 3 minutes until tender.
- Stir in flour, then whisk remaining broth until combined and cook soup or until thicken slightly, stirring constantly.
- Add cooked rice blend in the soup along with chicken and carrots, stir well and simmer for 5 minutes.
- Ladle soup into four bowls, garnish with parsley and almonds, and serve.

Nutrition Information –

287 Cal; 35 g Carb; 21 g Protein; 7 g Fat, 1.6 g Fiber; 182 mg Sodium; 384 mg Potassium; 217 mg Phosphorus;

Cauliflower Manchurian

|Preparation Time: 10 minutes|

|Cooking Time: 25 minutes|

|Total Time: 35 minutes|

|Serve – 6|

|Ingredients|

- 1 medium head of cauliflower, cut into florets
- ½ teaspoon minced garlic
- 1 teaspoon grated ginger
- 2 tablespoons rice flour
- 1/2 teaspoon red chili powder
- 1 teaspoon curry powder
- 1/2 teaspoon cumin powder
- 1 teaspoon lemon juice
- 4 cups canola oil

|Directions|

- Place cauliflower florets in a heatproof bowl, cover with plastic wrap, make holes in the wrap with a fork and microwave for 12 minutes

at medium heat setting until florets are steamed and softened, not mushy.
- Add rice flour into the florets along with garlic, ginger, red chili powder, curry powder, and cumin and stir until well coated.
- Place a deep frying pan over medium heat, pour in the oil, and when hot, add cauliflower florets in it in a single layer and cook for 5 minutes until golden brown.
- When done, drizzle lemon juice over the cauliflower and serve hot.

Nutrition Information –

77 Cal; 6 g Carb; 2 g Protein; 5 g Fat, 1.9 g Fiber; 23 mg Sodium; 225 mg Potassium; 36 mg Phosphorus;

Ratatouille

|Preparation Time: 10 minutes|

|Cooking Time: 50 minutes|

|Total Time: 60 minutes|

|Serve – 16|

|Ingredients|

- 2 cups diced zucchini squash
- 1 medium red bell pepper, cored, diced
- 3 cups diced yellow crookneck squash
- 1 medium yellow bell pepper, cored, diced

- 1 medium eggplant, diced
- 2 medium carrots, peeled, diced
- 1 medium green bell pepper, cored, diced
- 2 cups diced white onion
- 1 cup diced tomatoes
- 1 tablespoon fresh rosemary
- 2 teaspoons minced garlic
- 1 tablespoon fresh thyme
- 2 tablespoons olive oil
- 1 tablespoon fresh sage
- 1 tablespoon fresh basil
- 1 tablespoon freshly cracked black pepper
- 1 tablespoon fresh oregano
- 8 tablespoons grated parmesan cheese, sodium-reduced

|Directions|

- Take a large skillet pan, add oil and when hot, add carrot, garlic, black pepper, and all the herbs, then stir until mixed and cook for 2 minutes.
- Then add remaining ingredients, except for tomatoes and cheese, stir well, and cook for 15 minutes until vegetables are semi-tender.
- Add tomatoes and cheese into the pan, stir until well mixed and simmer for 30 minutes, covering the pan.
- Serve straight away.

Nutrition Information –

54 Cal; 6 g Carb; 3 g Protein; 3 g Fat, 2.4 g Fiber; 84 mg Sodium; 302 mg Potassium; 58 mg Phosphorus;

Roasted Brussels Sprouts, Carrots and Apples

|Preparation Time: 10 minutes|

|Cooking Time: 40 minutes|

|Total Time: 50 minutes|

|Serve – 8|

|Ingredients|

- 3 large carrots, peeled
- 20 medium Brussels sprouts, trimmed
- 2 medium apples, cored
- 1 teaspoon cinnamon
- 1/4 teaspoon salt
- 1/2 teaspoon nutmeg
- 2 tablespoons maple syrup
- 1/4 cup olive oil

|Directions|

- Switch on the oven, then set it to 375 degrees F and let it preheat.

- Meanwhile, cut each sprout into half, cut the carrot into 1-inch pieces, cut the apple into ½-inch cubes, and place them in a large bowl.
- Prepare the sauce and for this, stir together cinnamon, salt, nutmeg, maple syrup, and oil until combined, then pour the sauce over vegetables and apples in the bowl and stir until well coated.
- Take a baking sheet, grease it with oil, add prepared vegetables and apples on it, season with salt, and then bake for 40 minutes until form-tender.
- Serve straight away.

Nutrition Information –

140 Cal; 17 g Carb; 2 g Protein; 7 g Fat, 3.8 g Fiber; 105 mg Sodium; 332 mg Potassium; 48 mg Phosphorus;

Chicken Lettuce Wraps

|Preparation Time: 10 minutes|

|Cooking Time: 18 minutes|

|Total Time: 28 minutes|

|Serve – 4|

|Ingredients|

- 8 ounces chicken breast, cooked, mined
- 1/4 cup chopped red onion

- 1/4 cup chopped mushroom
- 2 scallions, chopped
- 1/4 cup chopped fresh cilantro
- 2 teaspoons minced garlic
- 1 teaspoon Chinese Five Spices seasoning
- 2 teaspoons hoisin sauce
- 2 tablespoons rice vinegar, unseasoned
- 2 tablespoons canola oil
- 1 tablespoon sesame oil
- 8 lettuce leaves

|Directions|

- Take a skillet pan, place it over medium heat, then add sesame oil and canola oil and when hot, add chicken, garlic and scallion, season with Chinese five spices, drizzle with vinegar and hoisin sauce and stir until mixed.
- Switch heat to medium-low level, cook for 15 minutes, stirring frequently, and then transfer chicken to a serving bowl.
- Prepare the lettuce wrap and for this, place a lettuce leaf on working space, top it with ¼ cup of cooked chicken mixture, top evenly with red bell pepper, mushroom, onion, and cilantro and then wrap the lettuce around the chicken.
- Preparing remaining lettuce wraps in the same manner and then serve.
-

Nutrition Information –

219 Cal; 4 g Carb; 17 g Protein; 15 g Fat, 0.8 g Fiber; 103 mg Sodium; 225 mg Potassium; 130 mg Phosphorus;

Chicken Parmesan Meatballs

|Preparation Time: 10 minutes|

|Cooking Time: 25 minutes|

|Total Time: 35 minutes|

|Serve – 10|

|Ingredients|

- 1 pound ground chicken
- 3 tablespoons breadcrumbs
- 1/4 teaspoon garlic powder
- 1/4 teaspoon onion powder
- 1/4 teaspoon Italian seasoning
- 1 tablespoon grated Parmesan cheese, sodium-reduced
- 1/2 cup shredded mozzarella cheese, sodium-reduced
- 1 pasteurized egg
- 8 ounces pizza sauce, low-sodium
- Cauliflower rice for serving

|Directions|

- Switch on the oven, then set it to 375 degrees F and let it preheat.
- Meanwhile, place chicken in a bowl, add 2 tablespoon pizza sauce, egg, parmesan cheese, breadcrumbs, and season with garlic powder, onion powder, and Italian seasoning.
- Stir until well mixed, shape the mixture into thirty small meatballs, arrange them on a baking sheet greased with oil and then bake for 15 minutes until cooked.
- Take a glass baking dish, spread some of the remaining pizza sauce in the bottom, arrange meatballs in the dish, top with remaining pizza sauce, sprinkle cheese on top and continue baking for 10 minutes.
- Serve meatballs with cooked cauliflower rice.

Nutrition Information –

114 Cal; 4 g Carb; 11 g Protein; 6 g Fat, 0.5 g Fiber; 223 mg Sodium; 350 mg Potassium; 132 mg Phosphorus;

Mexican Chicken Pizza

|Preparation Time: 10 minutes|

|Cooking Time: 18 minutes|

|Total Time: 28 minutes|

|Serve – 4|

|Ingredients|

- 2 cups diced roasted chicken breast
- 1 cup whole-kernel corn, no-salt-added
- 1/4 cup diced white onion
- 1/2 cup diced red bell peppers
- 4 teaspoons chopped fresh cilantro
- ½ teaspoon minced garlic
- 1/2 cup Monterey Jack cheese, sodium-reduced
- 2 tablespoons lime juice
- 4 flour tortillas, each about 6-inch

|Directions|

- Switch on the oven, then set it to 350 degrees F and let it preheat.
- Then take a baking sheet, grease it with oil, then arrange tortillas in it and bake for 10 minutes until edges of tortillas start to brown.
- When done, remove tortillas from the oven, stack, and press them down and set aside until required.
- Place a large skillet pan over medium-high heat, grease it with oil and when hot, add corn and cook for 1 minute or more until lightly charred.
- Add chicken, red peppers, onion, and garlic, stir well, continue cooking for 2 minutes until thoroughly heated, then remove the pan from heat and stir in line juice.

- Arrange tortillas on the baking sheet, top each tortilla with ¾ cup of chicken mixture, top with 2 tablespoons of Monterey Jack cheese, and bake for 2 minutes until cheese has melted.
- When done, sprinkle cilantro on tortillas and stir well.

Nutrition Information –

309 Cal; 31 g Carb; 26 g Protein; 9 g Fat, 2.1 g Fiber; 253 mg Sodium; 329 mg Potassium; 250 mg Phosphorus;

Pita Pizza

|Preparation Time: 10 minutes|

|Cooking Time: 20 minutes|

|Total Time: 30 minutes|

|Serve – 2|

|Ingredients|

- 2 pieces of pita bread, each about 6-inch
- 2 ounces ground pork
- 1/4 cup chopped onion
- 1 teaspoon minced garlic
- 1/4 cup chopped green bell pepper
- 1/2 teaspoon fennel seeds
- 1/4 teaspoon red pepper flakes

- 1/3 cup shredded mozzarella cheese, sodium-reduced
- 2 tablespoons tomato sauce

|Directions|

- Switch on the oven, then set it to 400 degrees F and let it preheat.
- Meanwhile, place a frying pan over medium heat, add pork, onion, bell pepper, garlic and fennel, season with red pepper flakes, stir until mixed and cook for 7 to 10 minutes until cooked.
- Then take a baking sheet, grease it with oil, arrange pita bread on it, sprinkle evenly with cooked pork mixture, spread with 1 tablespoon of tomato sauce, sprinkle with half of the mozzarella cheese and bake for 8 to 10 minutes until cheese is bubbly.
- When done, drizzle remaining tomato sauce on pizza and then serve.

Nutrition Information –

284 Cal; 34 g Carb; 16 g Protein; 10 g Fat, 1 g Fiber; 381 mg Sodium; 303 mg Potassium; 189 mg Phosphorus;

Tofu Stir Fry

|Preparation Time: 10 minutes|

|Cooking Time: 15 minutes|

|Total Time: 25 minutes|

|Serve – 4|

|Ingredients|

- 16 ounces extra-firm tofu, pressed, drain, cubed
- 1 cup broccoli florets
- 1/2 of medium red bell pepper, cut into strips
- ½ teaspoon minced garlic
- 2 teaspoons sugar
- 2 tablespoons cornstarch
- 1/8 teaspoon freshly cracked black pepper
- 1/8 teaspoon cayenne pepper
- 1 teaspoon garlic and herb seasoning blend
- 11/2 tablespoon lime juice
- 11/2 tablespoon soy sauce, reduced-sodium
- 11/2 tablespoon canola oil
- 1 tablespoon sesame oil
- 1/2 cup unseasoned breadcrumbs
- 1/2 teaspoon sesame seeds
- 2 egg whites
- 2 cups steamed long-grain white rice

|Directions|

- Place soy sauce in a small bowl, add sugar and lime juice, stir well, and set aside until required.
- Place egg whites, breadcrumbs, and corn starch into three separate bowls.
- Prepare tofu pieces and for this, coat a tofu piece in cornstarch, then dip into egg whites and dredge into breadcrumbs.
- Place a skillet pan over medium-high heat, add oil and when hot, add tofu pieces in a single layer and cook for 5 to 8 minutes until nicely browned and crunchy.
- Transfer tofu pieces to a plate lined with a paper towel, then add sesame oil, and when hot, add bell pepper and broccoli florets and stir-fry for 3 minutes until tender-crisp.
- Add garlic, season with black pepper, cayenne pepper, and herb seasoning blend, stir well and cook for 1 minute.
- Return tofu pieces into the pan, toss well until mixed and pour in prepared soy sauce mixture, sprinkle with sesame seeds, and toss until well coated.
- Remove pan from heat, distribute tofu and vegetables between four plates and serve.

Nutrition Information –

400 Cal; 45 g Carb; 19 g Protein; 16 g Fat, 2.7 g Fiber; 584 mg Sodium; 317 mg Potassium; 177 mg Phosphorus;

Mediterranean Pizza

|Preparation Time: 10 minutes|

|Cooking Time: 15 minutes|

|Total Time: 25 minutes|

|Serve – 12|

|Ingredients|

- 1 pizza crust
- 1 Roma tomato, sliced
- 1 teaspoon sliced garlic
- 10 basil leaves, sliced
- 1 tablespoon olive oil
- 3 ounces goat cheese, sodium-reduced

|Directions|

- Switch on the oven, then set it to 450 degrees F and let it preheat.
- Meanwhile, place pizza crust on a baking pan, coat it with oil, scatter with garlic slices and then cover with tomato slices.

- Sprinkle tomato with basil leaves, then top with cheese and bake for 15 minutes until pizza has cooked.
- When done, slice the pizza into wedges and serve.

Nutrition Information –

176 Cal; 18 g Carb; 7 g Protein; 0 g Fat, 8 g Fiber; 240 mg Sodium; 86 mg Potassium; 90 mg Phosphorus;

Penne Pasta with Asparagus

|Preparation Time: 10 minutes|

|Cooking Time: 12 minutes|

|Total Time: 22 minutes|

|Serve – 6|

|Ingredients|

- 8 ounces whole-wheat penne pasta, cooked
- 1 pound asparagus
- 3 teaspoons minced garlic
- 1/2 teaspoon freshly cracked black pepper
- 1/8 teaspoon red pepper flakes
- 2 teaspoons lemon juice
- 1/4 teaspoon Tabasco sauce
- 2 tablespoon unsalted butter
- 2 tablespoons olive oil
- 1/4 cup shredded Parmesan cheese

|Directions|

- Take a skillet pan, place it over medium heat, then add oil and butter and when the butter melts, add garlic and red pepper and cook for 3 minutes or until sauté.
- Then cut asparagus into 2-inch pieces, add to the skillet pan, season with black pepper, drizzle with lemon juice and Tabasco sauce, stir well and cook for 6 minutes until tender-crisp.
- Place pasta in a large bowl, top with cooked asparagus, toss until mixed, and then top with cheese.
- Serve straight away.

Nutrition Information –

258 Cal; 33 g Carb; 9 g Protein; 10 g Fat, 4.8 g Fiber; 93 mg Sodium; 258 mg Potassium; 168 mg Phosphorus;

Vegetarian Egg Fried Rice

|Preparation Time: 5 minutes|

|Cooking Time: 15 minutes|

|Total Time: 20 minutes|

|Serve – 6|

|Ingredients|

- 1 cup extra-firm tofu, pressed, drained, dice
- 1 cup diced white onion
- 1 cup sliced carrots
- 1/2 cup green peas
- 1/2 cup chopped green onions
- 1/2 cup chopped cilantro
- 1 teaspoon minced garlic
- 1 tablespoon grated ginger
- 1/4 teaspoon dry mustard
- 1 tablespoon soy sauce, reduced-sodium
- 3 tablespoons canola oil
- 6 pasteurized eggs, beaten
- 4 cups rice, cooked

|Directions|

- Take a skillet pan, place it over medium heat, then add 1 tablespoon oil, and when hot, pour in eggs and cook for 3 minutes until eggs are scrambled to the desired level.
- Transfer eggs to a plate, add remaining oil into the pan, and when hot, add onion, carrot, peas, ginger, garlic, mustard, and tofu and stir well.
- Cook for 8 to 10 minutes until carrots are softened, then add eggs and rice, drizzle with soy sauce and mix well.
- Remove pan from heat, top with green onions and cilantro, and serve.

Nutrition Information –

343 Cal; 37 g Carb; 15 g Protein; 15 g Fat, 3.2 g Fiber; 238 mg Sodium; 350 mg Potassium; 230 mg Phosphorus;

Vegetable Casserole Delight

|Preparation Time: 5 minutes|

|Cooking Time: 4 minutes|

|Total Time: 9 minutes|

|Serve – 2|

|Ingredients|

- 1/2 cup sliced green beans
- 1/2 cup sliced yellow summer squash
- 1/8 teaspoon freshly cracked black pepper
- 1/8 teaspoon paprika
- 1 teaspoon olive oil
- 8 ounces liquid egg whites

|Directions|

- Take a heatproof dish or microwave dish, grease it with oil, arrange green beans and squash slices around the edges of the dish, and then pour in liquid egg whites.
- Season with black pepper and paprika, cover the dish and microwave for 4 minutes at high heat setting until done, stirring once.

- Serve straight away.

Nutrition Information –

76 Cal; 5 g Carb; 14 g Protein; 0 g Fat, 1.5 g Fiber; 207 mg Sodium; 344 mg Potassium; 42 mg Phosphorus;

Macaroni and Cheese

|Preparation Time: 5 minutes|

|Cooking Time: 12 minutes|

|Total Time: 17 minutes|

|Serve – 4|

|Ingredients|

- 1 cup elbow pasta
- 4 ounces diced green chilies
- 1/4 teaspoon freshly cracked black pepper
- 5-ounces Pimento Cheese spread made with cream cheese

|Directions|

- Place a medium saucepan, half-full with water, over medium heat, bring it to boil, then add pasta and cook for 7 to 10 minutes until tender.
- Drain the pasta, transfer it to a bowl, add cheese spread and chilies and stir until well combined and cheese has melted.

- Garnish with black pepper and serve immediately.

Nutrition Information –

196 Cal; 25 g Carb; 6 g Protein; 8 g Fat, 1 g Fiber; 227 mg Sodium; 83 mg Potassium; 74 mg Phosphorus;

Salmon Burgers with Coleslaw

|Preparation Time: 10 minutes|

|Cooking Time: 10 minutes|

|Total Time: 20 minutes|

|Serve – 5|

|Ingredients|

- 15 ounces cooked salmon, each about 5 ounces, skinless, boneless
- 5 cups coleslaw mix
- 1/8 teaspoon onion powder
- 1/8 teaspoon cracked black pepper
- ½ teaspoon garlic and herb seasoning blend
- ¼ teaspoon dried dill
- ½ cup dry panko breadcrumbs, unseasoned
- 3 tablespoons white vinegar
- 1 pasteurized egg
- 1 pasteurized egg white
- 1 cup yogurt

|Directions|

- Place yogurt in a bowl, add garlic and herb seasoning, onion powder and vinegar, and whisk well until combined.
- Add coleslaw mix, stir until well mixed and then refrigerate until required.
- Place salmon in a bowl, break it into flakes by using two forks, add black pepper, dill and panko breadcrumbs, pour in egg white and egg, stir until well mixed and then shape the mixture into five patties.
- Take a large skillet pan, place it over medium heat, grease it with oil and when hot, add salmon patties and cook for 5 minutes per side until golden brown.
- Serve salmon patties with prepared coleslaw mix and serve.

Nutrition Information –

198 Cal; 14 g Carb; 23 g Protein; 4 g Fat, 1.8 g Fiber; 347 mg Sodium; 505 mg Potassium; 354 mg Phosphorus;

Honey Mustard Grilled Chicken

|Preparation Time: 5 minutes|

|Cooking Time: 15 minutes|

|Total Time: 20 minutes|

|Serve – 4|

|Ingredients|

- 1 pound chicken breasts, skinless
- 2 green onions, chopped
- 1 tablespoon honey
- 1 teaspoon apple cider vinegar
- 1 1/2 tablespoons mustard
- 1/3 cup mayonnaise

|Directions|

- Prepare sauce and for this, place all the ingredients in a bowl except for chicken and stir until well mixed, reserving ¼ cup of the sauce for later use.
- Set the grill over medium-high heat, brush the grilling rack with oil and when hot, place chicken breasts on it, brush with prepared sauce and grill for 10 to 12 minutes until thoroughly cooked, brushing with sauce and turning chicken breasts frequently.

- Serve grilled chicken breasts with reserved mustard sauce.

Nutrition Information –

282 Cal; 5 g Carb; 25 g Protein; 18 g Fat, 0.2 g Fiber; 224 mg Sodium; 241 mg Potassium; 197 mg Phosphorus;

Broiled Haddock with Cucumber Salsa

|Preparation Time: 10 minutes|

|Cooking Time: 25 minutes|

|Total Time: 35 minutes|

|Serve – 4|

|Ingredients|

- 1 pound haddock
- 1 small ear of corn
- 1/2 cup peeled, diced cucumber
- 1/4 cup diced red bell pepper
- ½ teaspoon minced garlic
- 1/4 cup diced red onion
- 3 tablespoons chopped cilantro
- 1/2 teaspoon onion powder
- 1/4 teaspoon cayenne pepper
- 1/2 teaspoon garlic powder

- 1/2 teaspoon freshly cracked black pepper
- 4½ tablespoons lime juice

|Directions|

- Switch on the broiler and then let it preheat.
- Meanwhile, set the grill over medium-high heat, add corn and cook for 7 to 10 minutes until grill marks are apparent.
- Then let the corn cool for 5 minutes, cut the kernels from the stalk by using a sharp knife, and set aside until required.
- Prepare salad and for this, place onion, red bell pepper and cucumber in a bowl, add garlic, cilantro and corn kernel, season with cayenne pepper, drizzle with 1 ½ tablespoon lemon juice, toss until well mixed and then refrigerate until required.
- Cut haddock into four fillets, each about 4-ounces, then score them lightly and season with onion powder, garlic powder, and black pepper.
- Take a baking sheet, line it with parchment sheet, place the prepared fillet on it, drizzle with remaining lemon juice and then broil for 15 minutes, or until fish is fork-tender and nicely golden brown.
- Serve straight away.

Nutrition Information –

126 Cal; 6 g Carb; 22 g Protein; 1 g Fat, 0.9 g Fiber; 80 mg Sodium; 466 mg Potassium; 232 mg Phosphorus;

Citrus Salmon

|Preparation Time: 10 minutes|

|Cooking Time: 20 minutes|

|Total Time: 30 minutes|

|Serve – 6|

|Ingredients|

- 24 ounces of salmon fillets
- 1 teaspoon minced garlic
- 1 teaspoon dried dill
- 1 tablespoon capers
- ¼ teaspoon cayenne pepper
- 1 tablespoon Dijon mustard
- 1 teaspoon dried basil leaves
- 11/2 tablespoons lemon juice
- 1 tablespoon unsalted butter
- 2 tablespoons olive oil

|Directions|

- Prepare the sauce, and for this, place all the ingredients in a small saucepan, except for

salmon, place it over medium heat, stir well and bring the mixture to boil.
- Then switch heat to the low level, cook the sauce for 5 minutes, and set aside until required.
- While sauce is cooking, set the grill, brush its grilling rack with oil and let preheat at the medium-high level.
- Place salmon on the large piece of foil, fold the edges, and then place the foil packet containing salmon on the grill.
- Brush salmon with prepared sauce generously and cook for 12 minutes until fork-tender, covering the grill.
- When done, transfer salmon to a cutting board, cut it into six portions, and serve.

Nutrition Information –

294 Cal; 1 g Carb; 23 g Protein; 22 g Fat; 0.2 g Fiber; 190 mg Sodium; 439 mg Potassium; 280 mg Phosphorus;

Honey Spice-Rubbed Salmon

|Preparation Time: 10 minutes|

|Cooking Time: 10 minutes|

|Total Time: 20 minutes|

|Serve – 4|

|Ingredients|

- 3 cups arugula
- 16 ounces salmon fillets
- 1/2 teaspoon garlic powder
- 3/4 teaspoon lemon peel
- 1/2 teaspoon freshly cracked black pepper
- 1 sprig of dill
- 3 tablespoons honey
- 2 tablespoons olive oil
- 1 teaspoon hot water

|Directions|

- Prepare the sauce, and for this, place lemon peel in a bowl, add garlic powder, black pepper, honey, and water and then whisk well.
- Prepared salmon, and for this, spread the sauce on both sides of salmon and then rub it into the fillets with hands covered with gloves.
- Take a skillet pan, place it over medium heat, add oil and when hot, add salmon fillets and cook for 4 minutes.
- Then switch heat to medium-low level, flip the salmon, cook for another 6 minutes until salmon is fork-tender, and then transfer to a plate.
- Top salmon fillets with arugula, garnish with dill and serve.

Nutrition Information –

323 Cal; 15 g Carb; 23 g Protein; 19 g Fat, 0.4 g Fiber; 66 mg Sodium; 454 mg Potassium; 261 mg Phosphorus;

Salmon Soup

|Preparation Time: 5 minutes|

|Cooking Time: 20 minutes|

|Total Time: 25 minutes|

|Serve – 8|

|Ingredients|

- 1 pound salmon, cooked
- 1/2 cup chopped celery
- 1 medium carrot, peeled, chopped
- 1/2 cup chopped white onion
- 1/8 teaspoon freshly cracked black pepper
- 1/4 cup cornstarch
- 2 tablespoons unsalted butter
- 2 cups coconut milk, unsweetened
- 1/4 cup water
- 2 cups chicken broth, low-sodium

|Directions|

- Place a large saucepan over medium-high heat, add butter and when it melts, add celery, carrot, and onion and cook for 5 to 7 minutes until tender.

- Cut salmon into chunks, add into the pan, season with black pepper, pour in the milk and chicken broth, stir well and bring the mixture to near-boil.
- Stir together cornstarch and water until mixed, slowly stir into the soup, switch heat to medium level and cook until soup has thickened to the desired level.
- Cook soup for 5 minutes, then ladle into bowls and serve immediately.

Nutrition Information –

155 Cal; 9 g Carb; 14 g Protein; 7 g Fat, 0.5 g Fiber; 113 mg Sodium; 369 mg Potassium; 218 mg Phosphorus;

Salmon Steaks with Herb Dressing

|Preparation Time: 10 minutes|

|Cooking Time: 18 minutes|

|Total Time: 28 minutes|

|Serve – 4|

|Ingredients|

- 2 pounds salmon steaks
- 1 medium white onion, peeled, sliced
- 1 tablespoon fresh chives
- 3 tablespoons chopped dill weed

- 1/2 teaspoon salt
- 10 whole black peppercorns
- 2 tablespoons chopped parsley
- 2 bay leaves
- 3/4 cup mayonnaise
- 1 ½ cup water
- 3 tablespoons buttermilk
- 1 lemon, juiced, zested
- 1 lemon, cut into wedges

|Directions|

- Prepare the dressing and for this, place mayonnaise in a bowl, add chives, lemon zest, 1 tablespoon lemon juice, 2 tablespoons dill, and buttermilk, stir until mixed and refrigerate for 1 hour, covering the bowl.
- Place a skillet pan, place it over medium heat, pour in water, add remaining lemon juice, along with onion, parsley, peppercorns, bay leaves, and salt, and stir until mixed.
- Bring the mixture to boil, then add salmon steaks, and simmer for 12 minutes until fork-tender, covering the pan.
- When done, remove the pan from heat, top salmon with prepared dressing, garnish with dill and serve with lemon wedges.

Nutrition Information –

398 Cal; 3 g Carb; 28 g Protein; 30 g Fat, 0.4 g Fiber; 391 mg Sodium; 515 mg Potassium; 309 mg Phosphorus;

Tuna Noodle Casserole

|Preparation Time: 10 minutes|

|Cooking Time: 25 minutes|

|Total Time: 35 minutes|

|Serve – 2|

|Ingredients|

- 1/2 cup frozen green peas
- 1/2 cup fresh sliced mushrooms
- 5 ounces cooked tuna, packed in water
- 1/4 cup dry breadcrumbs, unseasoned
- 1 tablespoon unsalted butter
- 1/2 cup sour cream
- 1/4 cup cottage cheese, sodium-reduced
- 2 ounces egg noodles, cooked

|Directions|

- Switch on the oven, then set it to 350 degrees F and let it preheat.
- Meanwhile, place tuna in a bowl, break it into flakes by using two forks, then add

mushrooms, peas, sour cream, and cheese and stir until combined.
- Add noodles into tuna mixture, stir until just mixed and then spoon it into a casserole dish, greased with oil.
- Place a skillet pan, add butter and when it melts, add breadcrumbs, stir well and cook for 3 minutes until slightly crunchy.
- Spread breadcrumbs mixture over the noodles and then bake the casserole for 20 minutes until the top is nicely browned.
- Serve straight away.

Nutrition Information –

415 Cal; 39 g Carb; 22 g Protein; 19 g Fat, 3.2 g Fiber; 266 mg Sodium; 400 mg Potassium; 306 mg Phosphorus;

Glazed Cornish Game Hen

|Preparation Time: 15 minutes|

|Cooking Time: 50 minutes|

|Total Time: 1 hour and 5 minutes|

|Serve – 2|

|Ingredients|

- 1 ¼ pound Cornish game hen, cleaned
- 1 teaspoon Dijon mustard

- 1 teaspoon Worcestershire sauce
- 3 tablespoons unsalted butter, melted
- 2 tablespoons apricot jam

|Directions|

- Switch on the oven, then set it to 375 degrees F and let it preheat.
- Meanwhile, prepare the hen and for this, clean its cavity by removing and discarding goblets, rinse the hen, and pat dry.
- Brush inside cavity of hen with 1 tablespoon of butter, place it over the baking sheet, and bake for 20 minutes.
- Meanwhile, prepare the glaze and for this, place remaining melted butter in a bowl, add mustard, apricot jam, and Worcestershire sauce and stir until well combined.
- After 20 minutes of baking time, brush the hen generously with prepared glazed and then continue baking for 30 minutes until the internal temperature of hen reaches 165 degrees F, basting hens with glaze every 10 minutes.
- When done, let the hen rest for 10 minutes, cut in half, and serve with remaining glaze.

Nutrition Information –

530 Cal; 20 g Carb; 29 g Protein; 37 g Fat, 0 g Fiber; 183 mg Sodium; 362 mg Potassium; 192 mg Phosphorus;

Cauliflower and Broccoli Mac-n-Cheese

|Preparation Time: 15 minutes|

|Cooking Time: 1 hour and 12 minutes|

|Total Time: 1 hour and 27 minutes|

|Serve – 8|

|Ingredients|

- 12 ounces penne pasta, uncooked
- 2 cups cauliflower florets
- 1/2 cup sliced onion
- 2 cups broccoli florets
- 3 tablespoons all-purpose white flour
- ½ teaspoon minced garlic
- 4 tablespoons unsalted butter
- 1/2 teaspoon freshly cracked black pepper
- 2 tablespoons spicy mustard
- 1/4 teaspoon nutmeg
- 1 cup panko-style breadcrumbs
- 21/2 cups rice drink
- 1/2 cup shredded parmesan cheese, sodium-reduced
- 1 cup shredded white cheddar cheese, sodium-reduced
- 1 cup shredded Swiss cheese, sodium-reduced

|Directions|

- Switch on the oven, then set it to 350 degrees F and let it preheat.
- Meanwhile, cook pasta and for this, place a medium saucepan, half-full with water, over medium heat, bring it to boil, then add pasta and cook for 7 minutes, set aside until required.
- In the meantime, place cauliflower and broccoli florets in a large bowl, cover it with plastic wrap, make holes in it by using a fork and microwave for 5 to 10 minutes until steamed, set aside until required.
- Then place a pot over medium heat, add 3 tablespoons butter and when it melts, add onion and garlic and cook for 4 minutes until tender.
- Stir in flour, then slowly whisk in milk until combined and then season with salt and black pepper.
- Continue cooking for 3 to 5 minutes until the mixture has thickened, add mustard, and then stir well.
- Place parmesan, cheddar, and swiss cheese in a bowl, then stir until well mixed, add 2/3 of the cheese mixture into the pot, stir well until cheese melts and remove the pan from heat.
- Drain the pasta, broccoli, and cauliflower, add to prepared cheese sauce and toss until well mixed.

- Take a 9 by 12 inches baking pan, grease it with oil, pour in mac and cheese mixture, then top with remaining cheese mix and baking for 30 minutes.
- Meanwhile, place a frying pan over medium heat, add remaining butter, and when it melts, add breadcrumbs, stir well and cook for 3 minutes.
- Then switch temperature of the oven to 400 degrees F, spread breadcrumbs mixture on top of casserole and continue baking for 10 minutes until top is browned.
- Serve straight away.

Nutrition Information –

442 Cal; 52 g Carb; 18 g Protein; 18 g Fat, 2.2 g Fiber; 308 mg Sodium; 278 mg Potassium; 315 mg Phosphorus;

Creamy Orzo and Vegetables

|Preparation Time: 10 minutes|

|Cooking Time: 24 minutes|

|Total Time: 34 minutes|

|Serve – 6|

|Ingredients|

- 1 cup orzo pasta, uncooked

- 1 medium carrot, peeled, shredded
- 1 small zucchini, chopped
- 1/2 cup frozen green peas
- 1 small onion, peeled, chopped
- ½ teaspoon minced garlic
- 1/4 teaspoon salt
- 1/4 teaspoon freshly cracked black pepper
- 1 teaspoon curry powder
- 2 tablespoons fresh parsley
- 2 tablespoons olive oil
- 3 cups chicken broth, low-sodium
- 1/4 cup grated Parmesan cheese, sodium-reduced

|Directions|

- Place a large skillet pan over medium heat, add oil and when hot, add onion, carrot, zucchini, and garlic, and cook for 5 minutes.
- Then season with salt and curry powder, pour in chicken broth, stir well and bring the mixture to a boil.
- Add pasta into the pan, stir well, bring the mixture to a boil, then switch heat to medium-low level and simmer for 10 minutes until pasta is tender and most of the liquid is absorbed, covering the pan.
- Then add peas, parsley, and cheese into the pasta, stir well and continue cooking for 4

minutes until vegetables are hot and pasta is creamy.
- Garnish pasta with black pepper and serve.

Nutrition Information –

176 Cal; 25 g Carb; 10 g Protein; 4 g Fat, 2.6 g Fiber; 193 mg Sodium; 170 mg Potassium; 68 mg Phosphorus;

Feta Pasta with Chicken and Asparagus

|Preparation Time: 10 minutes|

|Cooking Time: 15 minutes|

|Total Time: 25 minutes|

|Serve – 8|

|Ingredients|

- 16 ounces penne pasta, uncooked
- 8 ounces chicken breasts, skinless, cubed
- 1 pound asparagus spears, cut into 1-inch pieces
- 1/3 teaspoon garlic powder
- ½ teaspoon minced garlic
- 1/3 teaspoon freshly cracked black pepper
- 11/2 teaspoons dried oregano
- 5 tablespoons olive oil
- 1/4 cup crumbled feta cheese, sodium-reduced

- 1/2 cup chicken broth, low-sodium

|Directions|

- Place a medium saucepan, half-full with water, over medium heat, bring it to boil, then add pasta and cook for 7 to 10 minutes until tender.
- Meanwhile, place a large skillet pan over medium-high heat, add 3 tablespoons oil and when hot, add chicken pieces, season with ¼ teaspoon each of garlic and black pepper, stir and cook for 5 minutes until cooked and browned.
- When done, transfer chicken pieces to a plate lined with paper towels and set aside until required.
- Add asparagus and garlic into the pan, pour in the broth, season with oregano and remaining black pepper and garlic, and cook for 5 minutes until tender, covering the pan.
- Then return chicken into the skillet, cook for 3 minutes until warmed, add pasta and stir until well mixed.
- Remove pan from heat, let the cooked pasta sit for 5 minutes, then drizzle with remaining oil and stir until mixed.
- Sprinkle pasta with cheese and then serve.

Nutrition Information –

376 Cal; 49 g Carb; 18 g Protein; 12 g Fat, 3 g Fiber; 110 mg Sodium; 243 mg Potassium; 193 mg Phosphorus;

Creamy Shells with Peas and Bacon

|Preparation Time: 10 minutes|

|Cooking Time: 30 minutes|

|Total Time: 40 minutes|

|Serve – 6|

|Ingredients|

- 11/2 cups whole-wheat shell pasta, small, uncooked
- 3 slices of bacon
- 3/4 cup frozen green peas
- 1 cup sliced white onion
- 1 ½ teaspoon minced garlic
- 1/4 teaspoon freshly cracked black pepper
- 1 tablespoon lemon juice
- 2 tablespoons unsalted butter
- 1 tablespoon olive oil
- 1/2 cup grated Parmesan cheese
- 1 cup ricotta cheese, sodium-reduced, part-skim

- 16 cups water

|Directions|

- Place a large pot over medium-high heat, pour in water, and bring it to boil.
- Meanwhile, cut butter into pieces, then place it into a large bowl, add black pepper, butter, parmesan, and ricotta cheese, stir until mixed and set aside until required.
- Take a skillet pan, place it over medium heat, add oil and when hot, add bacon and cook for 7 to 8 minutes until crispy.
- Transfer bacon to a plate lined with paper towels, add onion into the pan, cook it for 3 minutes, then add garlic and cook for 1 minute until fragrant, set aside until required.
- Add pasta into boiling water, cook until slightly hard, then add peas and cook for 1 minute or more until pasta is tender.
- Drain pasta and peas, reserving 1 cup of cooking liquid, and set pasta and peas aside until required.
- Pour ½ cup of reserved pasta liquid into cheese mixture, add lemon juice, and then whisk well until smooth.
- Add peas and pasta, toss until well coated, pour in reserved liquid and stir well.
- Crumble the fried bacon, top it on pasta, sprinkle with additional black pepper, and serve.

Nutrition Information –

313 Cal; 27 g Carb; 13 g Protein; 14 g Fat, 3.3 g Fiber; 244 mg Sodium; 172 mg Potassium; 203 mg Phosphorus;

Hawaiian Rice

|Preparation Time: 5 minutes|

|Cooking Time: 10 minutes|

|Total Time: 5 minutes|

|Serve – 6|

|Ingredients|

- 2 cups brown rice, cooked
- 1/2 cup chopped red bell pepper
- 1/2 cup sliced mushrooms
- 1/2 cup pineapple chunks, in unsweetened juice
- 1/2 cup bean sprouts
- 1 teaspoon grated ginger root
- 1/4 teaspoon salt
- 1/2 tablespoon soy sauce, low-sodium

|Directions|

- Take a skillet pan, grease it oil, then heat it over medium heat and when hot, add bean sprouts, mushrooms, and bell pepper and cook for 5 minutes or until sauté.

- Then add remaining ingredients, except for rice, stir well and continue cooking for 3 minutes until thoroughly heated.
- Add mix, stir well until mixed and then serve immediately.

Nutrition Information –

97 Cal; 20 g Carb; 2 g Protein; 1 g Fat, 1.8 g Fiber; 135 mg Sodium; 181 mg Potassium; 67 mg Phosphorus;

Italian Style Vegetables and Pasta with Chicken

|Preparation Time: 5 minutes|

|Cooking Time: 18 minutes|

|Total Time: 23 minutes|

|Serve – 4|

|Ingredients|

- 2 ounces chicken, cooked, diced
- 1/4 cup chopped white onion
- 1/2 cup fresh broccoli florets
- 1/2 cup chopped green bell pepper
- 1/2 teaspoon garlic powder
- 1/8 teaspoon salt
- 1/4 teaspoon red pepper flakes
- 1 teaspoon dried rosemary

- 1 tablespoon fresh basil
- 1 tablespoon olive oil
- 2 teaspoons cornstarch
- 1/4 cup chicken broth, low-sodium
- 1 cup pasta twists, cooked

|Directions|

- Place a large frying pan over medium-high heat, add oil and when hot, add onion and broccoli florets and cook for 3 minutes until fried.
- Add garlic, rosemary, and basil, season with salt and red pepper, then add chicken and stir until mixed.
- Stir together cornstarch and chicken broth, add it into the pan, stir well and cook for 5 minutes until thickened.
- Add pasta, stir well and cook for 3 minutes until thoroughly warmed.
- Serve straight away.

Nutrition Information –

250 Cal; 28 g Carb; 15 g Protein; 9 g Fat, 3.7 g Fiber; 265 mg Sodium; 329 mg Potassium; 140 mg Phosphorus;

Dessert

Berry Galette

|Preparation Time: 10 minutes|

|Cooking Time: 30 minutes and 20 seconds|

|Total Time: 40 minutes and 20 seconds minutes|

|Serve – 6|

|Ingredients|

- 2 cups frozen mixed berries
- 1 refrigerated pie crust, unformed
- 21/2 tablespoons coconut sugar
- 1 tablespoon blackberry preserves

|Directions|

- Switch on the oven, then set it to 425 degrees F and let it preheat.
- Meanwhile, thaw the dough, then roll it into a 12-inch round and place it on a baking sheet greased with oil.
- Place mixed berries in a bowl, add 2 tablespoons sugar, and then stir well until combined.
- Then spread the mixture in the center of the dough, leaving 2 to 3 inches border, and fold the edges of the dough towards the filling, press gently to seal.

- Place blackberry preserve in a heatproof bowl, microwave for 20 seconds until melted, then brush on the fold in edges of the dough and bake for 10 minutes.
- Then switch temperature of the oven to 350 degrees F, continue baking for 20 minutes, and when done, sprinkle galette with remaining sugar.
- Cut galette into six wedges and serve.

Nutrition Information –

230 Cal; 33 g Carb; 2 g Protein; 10 g Fat, 3 g Fiber; 158 mg Sodium; 87 mg Potassium; 29 mg Phosphorus;

Berries Napoleon

|Preparation Time: 15 minutes|

|Cooking Time: 5 minutes|

|Total Time: 20 minutes|

|Serve – 6|

|Ingredients|

- 1/2 cup fresh raspberries
- 1/2 cup fresh blueberries
- 2 tablespoons brown sugar
- 1 tablespoon powdered swerve sugar
- 12 wonton wrappers
- 1 cup whipped topping, fat-free

|Directions|

- Switch on the oven, then set it to 400 degrees F and let it preheat.
- Meanwhile, taking a baking sheet, spray it with oil, spread wonton wrapper on it, and then spray them with oil.
- Sprinkle with sugar and then bake for 5 minutes until golden brown.
- When done, transfer six wonton wrappers on a serving tray, top each wrapper with 2 tablespoons whipped topping, 1 tablespoon each of berries, and then cover the top with another wrapper.
- Prepare the remaining Napoleon in the same manner, then sprinkle with swerve sugar and serve immediately.

Nutrition Information –

97 Cal; 20 g Carb; 2 g Protein; 1 g Fat, 1 g Fiber; 100 mg Sodium; 50 mg Potassium; 25 mg Phosphorus;

Banana Dessert

|Preparation Time: 3 hours and 10 minutes|

|Cooking Time: 10 minutes|

|Total Time: 3 hours and 20 minutes|

|Serve – 12|

|Ingredients|

- 7 ounces banana cream pudding mix
- 12 ounces vanilla wafers
- 8 ounces whipped topping
- 21/2 cups rice milk, unenriched

|Directions|

- Take a heatproof baking dish, about 9 by 13 inches in size, line it with wafer, and set aside until required.
- Place a saucepan over medium heat, add banana pudding mix, whisk in milk and bring the mixture to boil, stirring continuously.
- Evenly pour the pudding mixture over wafers, top with another layer of wafer, pressing into the pudding mixer, and then place it in the refrigerator for 1 hour until chilled.
- Spread whipped topping on top of the dessert, continue refrigerating for a minimum of 2 hours and serve.

Nutrition Information –

259 Cal; 46 g Carb; 3 g Protein; 7 g Fat, 0.3 g Fiber; 276 mg Sodium; 52 mg Potassium; 40 mg Phosphorus;

Crepes with Frozen Berries

|Preparation Time: 10 minutes|

|Cooking Time: 18 minutes|

|Total Time: 28 minutes|

|Serve – 4|

|Ingredients|

- 1/2 cup mixed frozen berries, thawed
- 1/2 cup all-purpose white flour
- 1 tablespoon powdered sugar
- 2 pasteurized egg whites
- 1 tablespoon canola oil
- 1/2 cup almond milk

|Directions|

- Place flour in a large bowl, add oil, egg whites, and milk and whisk until smooth.
- Take a skillet pan, place it over medium heat, grease it with oil, then pour in ¼ cup of prepared flour batter and spread it evenly by tilting the pan.
- Cook for 2 minutes, then flip the crepe, spoon 2 tablespoons of mixed berries in its center, and continue cooking for 2 minutes.
- Fold the cooked crepe in half, transfer it to a plate and dust with sugar.

- Use the remaining batter for cooking more crepes and then serving.

Nutrition Information –

124 Cal; 17 g Carb; 5 g Protein; 4 g Fat, 1.4 g Fiber; 41 mg Sodium; 123 mg Potassium; 55 mg Phosphorus;

Carrot Cake

|Preparation Time: 20 minutes|

|Cooking Time: 1 hour|

|Total Time: 1 hour and 20 minutes|

|Serve – 20|

|Ingredients|

- 2 cups all-purpose white flour
- 3 cups shredded carrots
- 1/2 teaspoon salt
- 1/2 teaspoon baking soda
- 2 tablespoons cinnamon
- 1 ¾ cup Splenda
- 1 teaspoon baking powder
- 1 teaspoon vanilla extract, unsweetened
- 1/2 cup unsalted butter
- 11/2 cups canola oil
- 4 pasteurized eggs
- 8 ounces softened cream cheese

|Directions|

- Switch on the oven, then set it to 350 degrees F and let it preheat.
- Place flour in a bowl, add baking powder, salt, baking soda, and cinnamon, stir well, and set aside until required.
- Place oil in another bowl, add 1 cup Splenda, whisk until combined, and then whisk in eggs, one at a time, until blended.
- Then whisk in flour mixture, ¼ cup at a time, until incorporated and then fold in carrot until combined.
- Take a heatproof baking dish, about 9 by 13 inches in size, grease it with oil, dust with flour, then pour in prepared batter, spread evenly, and bake for 60 minutes until the cake has cooked and inserted knife into the center of cake slide out clean.
- Meanwhile, prepare the icing and for this, place cream cheese in a bowl, add butter, beat well until combined and fluffy, and then beat in remaining Splenda and vanilla until combined.
- When cake has cooked, transfer it to a wire rack to cool completely, then spread with prepared icing, cut the cake into slices and serve.

Nutrition Information –

327 Cal; 17 g Carb; 4 g Protein; 27 g Fat, 1.2 g Fiber; 157 mg Sodium; 99 mg Potassium; 76 mg Phosphorus;

Stuffed Strawberries

|Preparation Time: 40 minutes|

|Cooking Time: 0 minutes|

|Total Time: 40 minutes|

|Serve – 12|

|Ingredients|

- 24 large strawberries
- 1/2 cup cream cheese, strawberry-flavored
- 3 tablespoons sour cream, reduced-fat

|Directions|

- Remove stems from strawberries and then rinse well.
- Prepare berries and for this, place a berry on a cutting board, point side up, then make a deep "X" in the top of the berry and then spread apart.
- Place cream cheese in a bowl, add sour cream, whisk well until beaten and smooth, and then pipe it into each strawberry.
- Refrigerate stuffed strawberries for 30 minutes until chilled and then serve.

Nutrition Information –

56 Cal; 4 g Carb; 1 g Protein; 4 g Fat, 0.8 g Fiber; 31 mg Sodium; 75 mg Potassium; 22 mg Phosphorus;

Sugarless Heart Cookies

|Preparation Time: 1 hour and 15 minutes|

|Cooking Time: 7 minutes|

|Total Time: 1 hour and 22 minutes|

|Serve – 12|

|Ingredients|

- 1 small box of mixed fruit gelatin, sugar-free
- 13/4 cups all-purpose white flour
- 1/2 teaspoon baking powder
- 1 teaspoon vanilla extract, unsweetened
- 3/4 cup unsalted margarine, softened
- 1/4 cup liquid egg substitute, low-cholesterol

|Directions|

- Switch on the oven, then set it to 400 degrees F and let it preheat.
- Meanwhile, place margarine in a bowl, add gelatin, beat until creamy and then beat in vanilla and egg substitute until blended.
- Place flour in another bowl, add baking powder, stir until mixed, and then slowly mix

into the margarine mixture until a smooth dough comes together.
- Place dough in a bowl, cover it with plastic wrap, and refrigerate for 1 hour until chilled.
- Then transfer the dough to a working space dusted with flour, roll it into a ¼-thick crust, and then cut out twenty-four cookies by using a heart-shaped cookie cutter.
- Take a baking sheet, arrange cookies on it, and then bake for 7 minutes until cookies are set and the bottom is lightly browned.
- When done, transfer cookies to a wire rack and let cool before serving.

Nutrition Information –

136 Cal; 14 g Carb; 2 g Protein; 8 g Fat, 0.5 g Fiber; 120 mg Sodium; 25 mg Potassium; 53 mg Phosphorus;

Low Phosphorus Fudge

|Preparation Time: 1 hour and 15 minutes|

|Cooking Time: 10 minutes|

|Total Time: 1 hour and 25 minutes|

|Serve – 18|

|Ingredients|

- 11/2 cups chocolate chips, semi-sweet

- 11/2 cups miniature-sized marshmallows
- 12/3 cups white sugar
- 1 teaspoon vanilla extract, unsweetened
- 2/3 cup half-and-half creamer

|Directions|

- Take a 9-inch square baking pan, grease it with oil, and set aside until required.
- Place a large saucepan over medium heat, add creamer and sugar, stir well and bring it to boil.
- Switch heat to medium-low level, continue boiling for 5 minutes, and then remove the pan from heat.
- Add vanilla, chocolate chips, and marshmallows into the pan, stir well until the marshmallow has melted, and then spoon the mixture immediately into the prepared baking span.
- Let the mixture cool until set, then cut it into eighteen pieces, each piece about 3 by 1 ½ inch in size , and then serve.

Nutrition Information –

177 Cal; 32 g Carb; 1 g Protein; 5 g Fat, 0.8 g Fiber; 10 mg Sodium; 64 mg Potassium; 27 mg Phosphorus;

Cherry Coffee Cake

|Preparation Time: 10 minutes|

|Cooking Time: 40 minutes|

|Total Time: 50 minutes|

|Serve – 24|

|Ingredients|

- 20 ounces cherry pie filling
- 2 cups all-purpose white flour
- 1 cup brown sugar
- 1 teaspoon baking powder
- 1 teaspoon baking soda
- 1 teaspoon vanilla extract, unsweetened
- 1/2 cup unsalted butter, softened
- 1 cup sour cream
- 2 pasteurized eggs

|Directions|

- Switch on the oven, then set it to 350 degrees F and let it preheat.
- Meanwhile, place flour in a bowl, add baking powder and baking soda and stir until mixed.
- Take another bowl, place remaining ingredients in it, except for cherry pie filling, whisk until blended and then slowly blend in flour mixture until incorporated and smooth.

- Take a heatproof 9 by 13 inches baking pan, grease it with oil, pour in prepared batter, then top with cherry pie filling and bake for 40 minutes until golden brown.
- Serve straight away.

Nutrition Information –

204 Cal; 30 g Carb; 3 g Protein; 8 g Fat, 0.5 g Fiber; 113 mg Sodium; 72 mg Potassium; 70 mg Phosphorus;

Cranberry and Apple Salad

|Preparation Time: 4 hours and 10 minutes|

|Cooking Time: 0 minutes|

|Total Time: 4 hours and 10 minutes |

|Serve – 10|

|Ingredients|

- 1 cup miniature-sized marshmallows
- 4 medium apples, cored, peeled
- 21/2 cups fresh cranberries
- 1/4 cup sugar
- 1 tablespoon fruit protector

|Directions|

- Place apples in a food processor, add cranberries and process until chopped.

- Tip the mixture into a bowl, top with fruit protection, mix well and then fold in marshmallows and sugar.
- Chill the salad for 4 hours, then stir and serve.

Nutrition Information –

64 Cal; 16 g Carb; 0 g Protein; 0 g Fat, 1.8 g Fiber; 2 mg Sodium; 66 mg Potassium; 9 mg Phosphorus;

Creamy Grape Salad

|Preparation Time: 1 hour and 10 minutes|

|Cooking Time: 0 minutes|

|Total Time: 1 hour and 10 minutes|

|Serve – 16|

|Ingredients|

- 3 pounds grapes, seedless, sliced vertically
- 1/2 cup sugar
- 2 teaspoons vanilla extract, unsweetened
- 8 ounces softened cream cheese
- 8 ounces sour cream

|Directions|

- Place cream cheese in a medium bowl, add sugar, vanilla, and sour cream and mix well until combined.

- Then add grapes, stir well until mixed and chill in the refrigerator for 1 hour.
- Serve straight away.

Nutrition Information –

168 Cal; 22 g Carb; 2 g Protein; 8 g Fat, 0.8 g Fiber; 58 mg Sodium; 202 mg Potassium; 48 mg Phosphorus;

Orange Pineapple Ambrosia Salad

|Preparation Time: 10 minutes|

|Cooking Time: 20 minutes|

|Total Time: 30 minutes|

|Serve – 4|

|Ingredients|

- 1/2 cup miniature-sized marshmallows
- 8 ounces crushed pineapple, in juice
- 8 maraschino cherries
- 11 ounces mandarin oranges
- 2 tablespoons grated coconut
- 1/4 cup sour cream

|Directions|

- Drain oranges and pineapple, then place them in a bowl and add remaining ingredients.

- Stir well until mixed and then place the salad in the refrigerator overnight until very chilled.
- Serve straight away.

Nutrition Information –

127 Cal; 24 g Carb; 1 g Protein; 3 g Fat, 1 g Fiber; 31 mg Sodium; 127 mg Potassium; 26 mg Phosphorus;

Caramel Custard

|Preparation Time: 45 minutes|

|Cooking Time: 45 minutes|

|Total Time: 1 hour and 30 minutes|

|Serve – 6|

|Ingredients|

- 3 cups coconut milk, unsweetened
- 1/2 cup and 4 tablespoons sugar
- 4 drops of vanilla extract, unsweetened
- 2 tablespoons water
- 6 pasteurized eggs

|Directions|

- Prepare caramel and for this, place 2 tablespoons sugar in a heatproof bowl, add 2 tablespoon water, stir well, and microwave for 4 minutes at high heat setting until sugar is caramelized.

- Then transfer caramel into a baking dish and let cool completely.
- Switch on the oven, then set it to 350 degrees F and let it preheat.
- Meanwhile, prepare the custard and for this, crack eggs in a bowl, beat until frothy, and then beat in vanilla.
- Gradually beat in remaining sugar and milk until combined, then top custard evenly on caramel and bake for 35 to 40 minutes until done.
- Cool the custard for 30 minutes until set, and then run a knife along the side of the baking dish.
- Place a serving dish on top of the baking dish, shake it and invert it to take out custard and then top with berries or fruit slices.
- Serve straight away.

Nutrition Information –

215 Cal; 29 g Carb; 9 g Protein; 7 g Fat, 6 g Fiber; 116 mg Sodium; 241 mg Potassium; 194 mg Phosphorus;

Pear Crisp

|Preparation Time: 10 minutes|

|Cooking Time: 45 minutes|

|Total Time: 55 minutes|

|Serve – 8|

|Ingredients|

- 3 pounds Asian pears, peeled, cored
- 1 lemon, juiced
- 1/2 cup all-purpose white flour
- 1/4 teaspoon ground cinnamon
- 1/4 cup brown sugar
- 4 tablespoons coconut sugar, divided
- 1/8 teaspoon ground nutmeg
- 3/4 cup chopped walnuts
- 1 tablespoon cornstarch
- 5 tablespoons unsalted butter

|Directions|

- Switch on the oven, then set it to 375 degrees F and let it preheat.
- Meanwhile, prepare the topping and for this, place flour in a bowl, add cinnamon, 2 tablespoon coconut sugar, brown sugar, nutmeg, and nuts, stir until mixed, and then slowly stir in butter until mixture resembles wet sand.

- Place remaining 2 tablespoons coconut sugar in a large bowl, add cornstarch and lemon juice and whisk well until combined.
- Peel and core each pea, then cut in half, add to sugar-corn starch mixture, toss until well coated, and then transfer pears into an 8-inch square baking dish.
- Sprinkle pears with prepared topping and then bake for 45 minutes until topping is nicely browned, and edges of pears are bubbling.
- When done, cool the prepared pear crisp on a wire rack and then serve.

Nutrition Information –

401 Cal; 56 g Carb; 6 g Protein; 15 g Fat, 12 g Fiber; 53 mg Sodium; 127 mg Potassium; 86 mg Phosphorus;

Dessert Pizza

|Preparation Time: 20 minutes|

|Cooking Time: 46 minutes|

|Total Time: 1 hour and 6 minutes|

|Serve – 8|

|Ingredients|

- 1 precooked pizza crust, about 12-inch
- 1 cup peaches
- 1 cup fresh sliced strawberry

- 5 tablespoons powdered sugar, divided
- 1/4 cup chocolate chips, unsweetened
- 1 cup ricotta cheese, sodium-reduced, part-skim
- 2 tablespoons warm jelly
- 1/2 cup apricot jam

|Directions|

- Switch on the oven, then set it to 425 degrees F and let it preheat.
- Meanwhile, strain cheese with a cheesecloth and set aside until required.
- Place apricot jam in a heatproof bowl and microwave for 1 minute at a high heat setting until it melts.
- Place a crust on a pizza pan, brush it with ham, then mix 3 tablespoon sugar and cheese and spread cheese mixture on top of the crust.
- Top ricotta cheese with peaches and berries, sprinkle with chocolate chips and remaining sugar and then bake for 10 minutes.
- When done, let pizza cool for 10 minutes, cut it into slices, and then serve.

Nutrition Information –

288 Cal; 49 g Carb; 8 g Protein; 6 g Fat, 18 g Fiber; 166 mg Sodium; 98 mg Potassium; 47 mg Phosphorus;

Something Extra – Snacks and Juices

Rhubarb Tea

|Preparation Time: 5 minutes|

|Cooking Time: 1 hour and 5 minutes|

|Total Time: 1 hour and 10 minutes|

|Serve – 8|

|Ingredients|

- 8 rhubarb stalks
- 1/3 cup sugar
- 8 cups of water
- ¼ cup mint leaves, to garnish

|Directions|

- Cut rhubarb stalks into 3-inch long pieces, then add them into a large pot and pour in water.
- Take the pot, place it over medium-high heat, bring the mixture to boil, then switch heat to medium level and simmer rhubarb for 1 hour.
- After 1 hour of cooking, strain the rhubarb liquid, then add sugar into the liquid, stir well and let cool completely.

- Distribute some ice into eight glasses, then pour in tea and serve.

Nutrition Information –

43 Cal; 11 g Carb; 0 g Protein; 0 g Fat, 2 g Fiber; 2 mg Sodium; 147 mg Potassium; 7 mg Phosphorus;

Lemonade

|Preparation Time: 35 minutes|

|Cooking Time: 0 minutes|

|Total Time: 35 minutes|

|Serve – 5|

|Ingredients|

- 5 cups lemon juice, fresh
- 5 cups of corn syrup

|Directions|

- Pour lemon juice in a pitcher, add corn syrup and stir until mixed.
- Then chill the lemonade in the refrigerator for 30 minutes and serve.

Nutrition Information –

98 Cal; 27 g Carb; 0 g Protein; 0 g Fat, 9 g Fiber; 40 mg Sodium; 32 mg Potassium; 2 mg Phosphorus;

Ginger and Cranberry Punch

|Preparation Time: 40 minutes|

|Cooking Time: 20 minutes|

|Total Time: 1 hour|

|Serve – 4|

|Ingredients|

- 1/3 cup coconut sugar
- 1/2 cup ginger, peeled, sliced
- 1/3 cup lime juice
- 4 cups cranberry juice

|Directions|

- Take a large pan, place it over medium heat, add ginger, pour in cranberry juice, and stir until mixed.
- Cook for 20 minutes, then add sugar and lime juice and stir well until sugar has dissolved.
- Strain the punch, let it cool for 30 minutes, and then serve.

Nutrition Information –

124 Cal; 31 g Carb; 0 g Protein; 0 g Fat, 10 g Fiber; 0 mg Sodium; 50 mg Potassium; 1 mg Phosphorus;

Raspberry Punch

|Preparation Time: 10 minutes|

|Cooking Time: 0 minutes|

|Total Time: 10 minutes|

|Serve – 24|

|Ingredients|

- 10 ounces frozen red raspberries, thawed
- 16 ounces raspberry sorbet
- 6 ounces pink lemonade concentrate, frozen
- 46 fluid ounces pineapple juice
- 8 ½ cups ginger ale, diet, chilled

|Directions|

- Take a large punch bowl, add ginger ale, raspberry sorbet, raspberry juice, and pineapple juice and stir until mixed.
- Then stir in raspberries until just combined, distribute between twenty-four cups and serve.

Nutrition Information –

70 Cal; 16 g Carb; 1 g Protein; 0 g Fat, 1.1 g Fiber; 8 mg Sodium; 91 mg Potassium; 6 mg Phosphorus;

Watermelon Summer Cooler

|Preparation Time: 5 minutes|

|Cooking Time: 0 minutes|

|Total Time: 5 minutes|

|Serve – 2|

|Ingredients|

- 1 cup watermelon cubes, seedless
- 1 tablespoon sugar
- 2 teaspoons lime juice
- 2 watermelon wedges, for garnish
- 1 cup crushed ice

|Directions|

- Place all the ingredients in a food processor or blender except for melon and pulse for 30 seconds until blended.
- Distribute the mixture between two glasses, garnish each glass with a watermelon wedge and serve.

Nutrition Information –

52 Cal; 13 g Carb; 0 g Protein; 0 g Fat, 0.3 g Fiber; 1 mg Sodium; 96 mg Potassium; 9 mg Phosphorus;

Spiced Almonds and Cashews

|Preparation Time: 10 minutes|

|Cooking Time: 15 minutes|

|Total Time: 25 minutes|

|Serve – 5|

|Ingredients|

- 1/2 cup almonds
- 1/4 teaspoon onion powder
- 1/8 teaspoon cayenne pepper
- 1/2 cup cashews
- 1/4 teaspoon garlic powder
- 1/4 teaspoon ground cumin
- 1/2 teaspoon Worcestershire sauce
- 1 tablespoon soy sauce, low-sodium

|Directions|

- Switch on the oven, then set it to 300 degrees F and let it preheat.
- Then take a baking sheet, spread almonds and cashews on it and bake for 10 to 15 minutes until cashews are golden brown.
- In the meantime, prepare the dressing and for this, place remaining ingredients in a bowl, whisk until combined, and set aside until required.

- When nuts have roasted, add them to the dressing and toss until well coated.
- Return nuts onto the baking sheet, continue cooking for 5 minutes, and then serve.

Nutrition Information –

164 Cal; 7 g Carb; 5 g Protein; 0 g Fat, 14 g Fiber; 61 mg Sodium; 183 mg Potassium; 135 mg Phosphorus;

Sweet Potato Fries

|Preparation Time: 5 minutes|

|Cooking Time: 15 minutes|

|Total Time: 20 minutes|

|Serve – 4|

|Ingredients|

- 2 large sweet potatoes, peeled

|Directions|

- Switch on the oven, then set it to 500 degrees F and let it preheat.
- Meanwhile, slice the sweet potatoes, then cut them into 1/8-inch pieces and place them on a greased baking sheet.
- Spray sweet potatoes with oil, and bake for 15 minutes until cooked and nicely golden brown.
- Serve straight away.

Nutrition Information –

68 Cal; 15 g Carb; 1 g Protein; 1 g Fat, 0 g Fiber; 8 mg Sodium; 132 mg Potassium; 18 mg Phosphorus;

Eggplant French Fries

|Preparation Time: 10 minutes|

|Cooking Time: 8 minutes|

|Total Time: 18 minutes|

|Serve – 6|

|Ingredients|

- 1 medium eggplant
- 3 teaspoons Ranch salad dressing seasoning Mix
- 3/4 cup cornstarch
- 1 teaspoon Tabasco sauce
- 3/4 cup dry bread crumbs, unseasoned
- 1/2 cup canola oil
- 2 pasteurized eggs
- 1 cup almond milk, unsweetened

|Directions|

- Peel and cut the eggplant into ¾-inch thick and 4-inch long stick, rinse well and then pat dry with paper towels.

- Pour milk in a bowl, add eggs, whisk until blended and then stir in hot sauce until mixed.
- Place breadcrumbs in a shallow dish, add cornstarch and ranch seasoning mix, and stir until mixed.
- Prepare eggplant fries and for this, dip the sticks into the egg mixture and then dredge into bread crumb mixture until evenly coated.
- Take a frying pan, pour in the oil, and when hot, add eggplant sticks and cook for 3 minutes per side until golden brown.
- When done, transfer eggplant sticks to a plate lined with paper towels and then serve.

Nutrition Information –

233 Cal; 24 g Carb; 5 g Protein; 13 g Fat, 2.1 g Fiber; 212 mg Sodium; 215 mg Potassium; 86 mg Phosphorus;

Zucchini French Fries

|Preparation Time: 10 minutes|

|Cooking Time: 8 minutes|

|Total Time: 18 minutes|

|Serve – 6|

|Ingredients|

- 2 medium zucchini

- 3/4 cup dry breadcrumbs, unseasoned
- 3 teaspoons Ranch salad dressing seasoning Mix
- 3/4 cup cornstarch
- 1 teaspoon Tabasco sauce
- 2 pasteurized eggs
- 1/2 cup canola oil
- 1 cup almond milk

|Directions|

- Peel and cut zucchini into ¾-inch thick and 4-inch long stick, rinse well and then pat dry with paper towels.
- Pour milk in a bowl, add eggs, whisk until blended and then stir in hot sauce until mixed.
- Then take a shallow dish, add breadcrumbs in it, then add cornstarch and ranch seasoning mix, and stir until mixed.
- Prepare zucchini fries and for this, dip the sticks into the egg mixture and then dredge into bread crumb mixture until evenly coated.
- Take a frying pan, pour in the oil, and when hot, add zucchini sticks and cook each side for 4 minutes until golden brown.
- When done, transfer zucchini sticks to a plate lined with paper towels and then serve.

Nutrition Information –

252 Cal; 22 g Carb; 5 g Protein; 16 g Fat, 1 g Fiber; 216 mg Sodium; 263 mg Potassium; 105 mg Phosphorus;

Thyme Corn on the Cob

|Preparation Time: 10 minutes|

|Cooking Time: 20 minutes|

|Total Time: 30 minutes|

|Serve – 4|

|Ingredients|

- 4 half-ear size corn on the cob, frozen
- 1/4 teaspoon freshly cracked black pepper
- 1/2 teaspoon dried thyme
- 2 tablespoons olive oil
- 1 tablespoon grated parmesan cheese, sodium-reduced

|Directions|

- Place thyme and black pepper in a small bowl, add cheese and oil, and stir until well mixed.
- Coat corn with the prepared oil mixture until thoroughly coated, place them in the center of a large aluminum foil sheet, then top corn with two ice cubes and make a packet by folding the top and ends, leaving some space for heat to circulate in the packet.
- Preheat the grill at high heat setting, then place corn packet on it and cook for 20 minutes until done, flipping corn halfway through.

- Serve straight away.

Nutrition Information –

125 Cal; 15 g Carb; 2 g Protein; 8 g Fat, 1.8 g Fiber; 26 mg Sodium; 188 mg Potassium; 63 mg Phosphorus;

Conclusion

Food is not just 'fuel for your body;' it becomes a part of you. You are what you eat, so foods do affect your health. When you have chronic kidney disease, one way to protect or slow down the loss of kidney function is a take a fresh look at the foods you eat. Share it with your doctor or dietician and see if your meal plan needs some alternations. Most of the patients with kidney diseases, at any stage, can get essential nutrients and vitamins by following a healthy, clean, and well-balanced diet. But if you are at the end stage of kidney disease or kidney failure, you will need to develop a special diet. For this, you will need to consult a specially trained renal dietician and work with him/her to create a plan to maintain the health of your kidneys. These changes in your diet will also reduce the risk of hypertension, heart attack, and stroke. Once you know what foods are right for you, you can make your own collection of kidney-friendly meals.

Bon Appetit!

www.ingramcontent.com/pod-product-compliance
Lightning Source LLC
Chambersburg PA
CBHW060825220526
45466CB00003B/982